# UNDER THE BRIDGE BACKWARDS

It takes courage to be a caregiver. It is also takes courage to write with unflinching honesty the story of your family as you face an Alzheimer's diagnosis together. Barbara Roy fills her memoir with the highs and lows of many adjustments and altered expectations. She lets the reader accompany her, her husband, Phil, and their family on their voyage through Alzheimer's.

> — Ted Bowman, author of *Loss of Dreams: A Special Kind of Grief* and *Finding Hope When Dreams Have Shattered*

I recommend this book to all caregivers and families of patients with memory problems or Alzheimer's disease. From first encountering problems at home to reluctantly acknowledging that it's acceptable to ask family and friends for assistance, it will help readers deal with a surprising variety of challenges. It is full of wisdom that will provide much needed perspective to caregivers and especially those who support them.

> — Charles Ormiston, MD, board certified neurologist in private practice

Poetically written with compassion, honesty, and grace, this book will inform and support the tumultuous journey of caregivers and the people who care about them. Fellow clinicians and all others who give care to one who suffers from Alzheimer's disease or their family members will be glad to have found this insightful personal story.

> — Abby Dawkins, MSW, LICSW, Clinical Social Worker

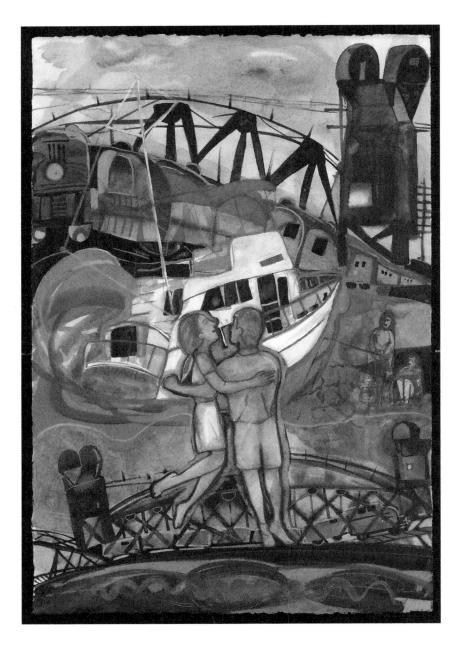

*Memories: Dances, Dreams, and Deliverance*

# UNDER THE BRIDGE BACKWARDS

## My Marriage, My Family, and Alzheimer's

**Barbara Blanch Roy**

 7T
BOOKS

*for Phil,*
*who gave me laughter and tears*

He who hears the rippling of rivers . . . will not utterly despair.
—Henry David Thoreau

# Contents

# CHAPTER 1

# Tying Knots

*Everyone to whom much was given, of him much will be required.*

— LUKE 12:48

This familiar Bible verse has always been a cautionary tale for me. Steeped in blessings, I have wondered, "What might be required of me?" On the other hand, I ask, "Where do all my blessings come from?" I'm inclined to accept them, say, "Thank you, God," and enjoy the abundance. I believe that the joy of swimming in blessed waters with loving family and trusted friends is not conditional. It's not a gift with strings. I do not accuse God in our misfortune of Alzheimer's. Perhaps science will one day explain how the disease infected the brain of my beloved husband, Phil. We most certainly did face difficult requirements in its clutches, but blessings did not run off.

Phil and I married in 1964, while he was still in medical school. When we became engaged, Phil's mother warned me that medical marriages are tough. Phil's father and grandfather had been doctors. I listened politely, imagining I could weather the demands. Phil's critical work in patient care was important to me too. I was proud of him and glad he would be helping others.

I was also naive. Early starts to long surgical days, weekends of being on call, hospital calls in the middle of the night, patient calls in the middle of dinner, medical meetings mixed up with vacations: all diverted

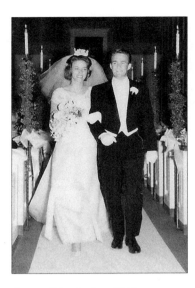

*Our wedding in June 1964*

his attention from our family. These demands were hard on Phil, me, and our four children. None of us were whiners. We loved each other and did our best to carry on.

In 1973, we bought an old summerhouse on the scenic St. Croix River as an antidote to medical practice, a recreational getaway for our family. A wide grassy plateau between the beach and the house served as a ball field. A large, screened porch wrapped around the front of the 1902 house, accommodating wet bathing suits, sandy feet, and the breeze off the river. Fortunate in having such an amazing place, I wanted to share it with others. "Come out to the river" was an easy invitation. Friends often brought food. We swam, played tennis, piled onto our pontoon boat, and relaxed. Our sturdy brick house, the hospitals, and the children's school remained in St. Paul.

Off-call, Phil drew us into project mode on our eight acres of riverfront land. He'd pull on a worn-out sweatshirt and faded jeans and call our young family to attention. When he ordered two hundred Norway pine seedlings from the state's Department of Natural Resources, he tied knots at ten-foot intervals in a long rope to show us where we should dig the planting holes. An infestation of Dutch elm disease gave him the excuse to buy his first chainsaw. An early riser, Phil started the racket before the neighbors were awake. The children's reward for picking up all the branches he downed was to have a turn driving the tractor and pulling the trailer of brush to his fire pit. Together we pitched the debris in and returned for more loads. For the dramatic last step, the children and I stood back, and Phil torched the pile. He loved having helpers and giving direction. I believed in family team effort, physical work, and fresh air.

The simple life of wet suits and small sandy feet disappeared when we built a lovely, year-round home next to the summerhouse in 1983. At the same time, Phil lost his troops. Our conscripted adolescents chafed: "Dad, we can't even invite our friends out to the river; all you want us to do is work!" They created imaginative excuses and offered legitimate reasons to absent themselves.

The new house was Phil's and my dream creation. Its architecture suited the site. The open interior spaces echoed the outdoors. Expansive glass made the river view an important feature in most rooms. A screened porch and multiple decks delivered us to manicured gardens. Phil and I still enjoyed working outdoors, but we had to hire a lawn service because we could no longer manage the landscaped property on our own.

At the same time we were building our new house, Phil had insisted on making a real estate investment in a loft apartment complex in downtown St. Paul. Facing the new farmer's market, the Market House was to be a cornerstone of Mayor Latimer's city development. Phil saw little risk and a tax break. I was skeptical primarily because he had no business experience. His surgical practice was booming, we were building our own house, and scant family time was disappearing. I begged him to skip the investment opportunity. When he ignored my reasoning and pleas, I had the project attorney create a document that held me harmless. All the partners signed it.

Phil's involvement with his big investment made him busier than ever in the city, away from the river. Our two oldest daughters attended private school in town, leaving our two youngest children and me to enjoy the country life with pristine snow and animal tracks. When our

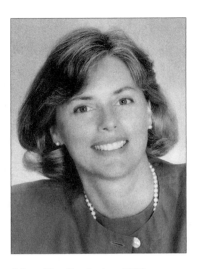

*Me at First Bank, circa 1988*

third daughter elected to attended her sisters' school in town for seventh grade, I joined the exodus and accepted a position in public affairs at First Bank St. Paul. Our youngest child, Christopher, in second grade, adjusted to the neighbor woman I hired to greet him after school and fix a snack.

Our house construction had gone over budget, interest rates were at 18 percent, and the Market House project was teetering. I wanted to contribute to our financial security and felt ready to translate my considerable volunteer experience into employment. Phil seemed pleased with my contributions to the family purse and my community accomplishments. I enjoyed working with corporate leaders and having a life independent of family responsibilities. My corporate duties kept increasing as I was promoted in a rapidly changing banking environment that eventually landed me in downtown Minneapolis.

With Phil embroiled in a failing Market House project and me sucked into a troubled workplace, we had less time to enjoy each other and our home's beautiful setting. We didn't pay enough attention to our own relationship and relied too little on the restorative powers of river life. We were foolish, stuck in our own mess.

In 1993 I left the bank. The depth of the Market House failure was known; our resulting debts were largely paid off. Phil and I were grateful to have survived our absence from one another and thrilled to witness new marital promises by our daughter Heidi and her neighborhood sweetheart, Rob. Event planners erected a white tent on our lawn; the florist decorated tent poles and dining tables. Music played, friends danced, and the river glistened approvingly. How lucky we all were!

When Phil retired five years later, we were finally able to put our marriage before medicine. We divided our property again and built a smaller, one-story house in 1999. Nestling it into a natural tallgrass prairie, we planted wildflowers and anticipated their reseeding. We had so much less to take care of! Though we no longer had a river view, we easily walked there on our narrow easement between the summerhouse and the big riverfront house. We were delighted to live more simply and less expensively, still on part of our original eight acres.

We had weathered economic inflation and marital storm. We'd applied hard work and joint problem solving. We'd suffered the humbling effect of life's challenges and our own insufficiency. In all, our marital knot had held.

# CHAPTER 2

# Letting Go

Paddling a canoe on the St. Croix River, Phil planted his first kiss on me. I was nineteen, home from college for the summer. He was to enter the University of Minnesota Medical School in the fall. We had jobs but also plenty of time to play. One hot summer day, we borrowed his dad's big portable radio, packed some snacks, and headed to the town of Taylors Falls to rent a canoe. The water sparkled in the bright sunlight. We glided easily along in the calm current until suddenly the bow where I sat lurched down. I turned around in alarm, only to find Phil crouching immediately behind me. Eyes dancing, he pulled me to him and delivered his kiss. We almost flipped. Food flew. The radio nearly went overboard. I was both startled and charmed. He quickly climbed back to the stern, the canoe steadied, and the river conspired to carry us on.

I am thankful for that day, my man, and the river, which continued to inform our lives in remarkable ways. After Heidi and Rob's 1993 summer wedding, his parents invited us to cruise the St. Croix on their Grand Banks trawler, *Summer Song*. Phil and I were entranced with its beauty. Its handsome outline was trimmed in shining teak. The well-designed galley and staterooms were efficient and comfortable. Plying the water slowly, we spent an idyllic evening. Rob's father, Stan, could see our pleasure. "Why wait? Get one now," he said.

The river was offering us a way forward after our long, hard recovery from the Market House debacle. A costly boat worried me. Still, a

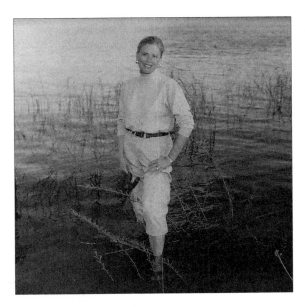

*Me enjoying the river, 1993*

boat would be an investment in spending time together. I backed off my financial caution and began to imagine the possibility with real interest. Phil was already ahead of me.

He contacted a boat dealer who found a used Grand Banks in Naples. Next he called my boat-owner father in Florida and asked him to go with him to inspect the trawler. Away he flew, picking up Dad and driving to Florida's west coast. The deal was made; arrangements to truck the thirty-six-foot boat to nearby Windmill Marina followed. We were boat owners!

Buying a boat wouldn't automatically solve our need for joint endeavor. The key would be committing to use it. Our first step was to choose its name together. We agreed on *Argonauta*. We embraced both the image of the delicate shell that small squid-like creatures cast away when they launch their young and the story of Jason's harrowing adventure that returned him home safely (but never to become king). We put ourselves on notice. The boat would be a commitment to a new way of life, with few parental responsibilities and without chasing the Golden Fleece.

When marina staff called in November to announce our boat's arrival, I reeled in a swirl of excitement and reservation. Was this wild jump lunacy? I raced to the marina to watch the truck unloading. Phil hurried home from the hospital and drove directly to meet me there. With the flying bridge dismantled and the mast secured horizontally, our boat did not resemble the beautiful *Summer Song*. But we were smitten like parents of a newborn babe.

Over the winter of 1994 the marina staff reassembled our boat and redid the brightwork. Also, Phil's blood pressure was way up. He made an appointment to see David Bartsch, a medical colleague, for advice. The morning of the appointment I called David myself. I'd felt in such a box because, at Phil's request, I'd not spoken to anyone about his health. When David came on the line, I burst into tears. My emotions tumbled out, and I felt such relief that I had to compose myself to speak. He was grateful for my call. I told him to tell Phil I'd called if he wanted to, but that I simply had to reveal my concern for Phil's well-being.

The good news was that Phil's physical issues were not life threatening. The further good news was that they talked about stress and emotional health. David broached the delicate topic of balancing hard work and taking good care of oneself. Phil told me afterwards that he was even considering counseling to alleviate his "demons." In my mind, no one had worked harder or tried harder to do what he thought was expected of him. My partner was a weary performer occasionally plagued by disappointment in himself. He needed to give himself a break. I was thankful for his trust in allowing me to see his vulnerability. With proper medication and some soul baring, he felt better. Unsurprisingly, he did not try counseling at that time.

Phil's sense of humor often saved him. Weeks later he came home hobbling after a long day of surgery. Something was hurting his foot. I looked at him sympathetically and offered, "I wish there was a way to cut off everything that doesn't work." In quick response he said with a twinkle, "All I'd have left would be my asshole!" In exhaustion and discomfort, he chose to laugh at himself and accept a hug.

By April the *Argonauta* was in the water hooked up to shore power. Phil and I began the interior cleaning enthusiastically. The shop manager in the marina gave us operating lessons in preparation for our maiden voyage. On a windless, blue-sky afternoon, we set out. I threw the lines on the dock, and Phil slowly backed out of the slip. Using the twin screws, he turned the bow toward the marina entrance and followed the buoys out to open water. We were happy rookies.

I took the wheel while Phil tended flapping canvas and checked various gauges. Soon we were snuggled side by side on the broad captain's bench, watching the shoreline that led to our house. Our carefully manicured property looked back at us and then slid from view as we absentee landlords swung past the sand bar at St. Mary's Point and crossed to the Wisconsin cove area. A few speedboats with water skiers zoomed past us, reminding me of the days I pulled our young children behind a small runabout. Soon we approached the no-wake zone at Catfish Bar and turned back to the marina.

Our first big adventure a few weeks later was an overnight trip downriver to Red Wing, which meant handling the lift bridge at Prescott and then Lock and Dam No. 3 on the Mississippi River. I provisioned the boat with food, bedding, clothes, CDs, and books. Phil double-checked

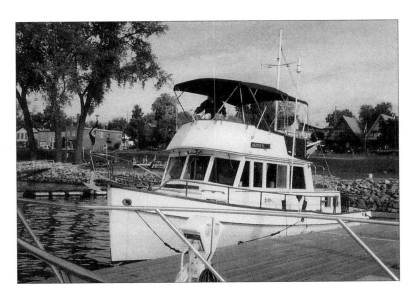

*The* Argonauta *tied up at Pepin, Wisconsin*

the engine room and measured the diesel fuel levels with a long dowel. Within two hours of leaving the marina, we saw the lift bridge at the confluence of the St. Croix and Mississippi Rivers. I called the bridge master on the ship's radio requesting southbound passage into the Mississippi. He called back announcing a ten-minute delay, as a train was due to cross.

As we waited in neutral, the current pushed us forward awkwardly. The boat swung left and then right in the wind. Phil reversed one engine and then the other to straighten our wobbly course. We were getting ever closer to the bridge, and then the engines cut out all together! By this time, the train was on the bridge but not fully across. Bobbing in a boat with no power, I watched in horror as the last cars went by. The bridge went up. We careened under it, swept backwards into the Mississippi River, and drifted perilously close to the rocky shore where Hmong fishermen stood with their poles.

Phil and I had no experience in maintaining power at idle. I was wide-eyed, dumbfounded, and shaken. If we had crashed, our beautiful boat would have been ruined. If we'd hurt the fishermen, I couldn't have forgiven myself. I didn't even imagine that we might have been injured.

The current carried us safely into the Big Muddy. On our ship radio the bridge master spoke flatly, "I've never seen a passage quite like that." I was giddy with relief. We'd survived our own ineptitude. Only then did I remember our son-in-law's caution not to cut the engines back too far, as they would die. I suggested to Phil that he simply restart them. He did with a smile, and we proceeded on our way.

Resuming, we were not afraid to face the lock at Red Wing. Rather, I felt buoyant in a wonderful, new way. Stripped of old recriminations, disappointments, and unmet expectations, I embraced our new adventure together. Phil had not succumbed to anger. I couldn't put words to it at the time, but I savored the mysterious, transformative moment. A precious intimacy was born in the emotional trauma of our near mishap. Being out of control had not mattered. A gracious current had protected us.

In the past, I had not taken mishap lightly. In fact, I had spent my whole life in an urgent effort toward responsibility—toward anything that I might do to improve a situation, like trying to make a difference, knowing what might be needed, doing my best, helping others to do their best, avoiding stupid mistakes, being prudent, and trying to remember to summon God's help. I had never intended to be arrogant or judgmental, but the truth was that pride had slipped into me from time to time, inviting those love-squelching behaviors. Floating safely in the river, I knew God's unbidden love was there for us.

Our time on board the *Argonauta* was full of mutual appreciation, honesty, and deep sharing—all of which were essential for the Alzheimer's voyage to come. The experience of going under the bridge backwards reinforced the importance of letting go and finding a new way of doing things together. Our conscious decision to embrace change had paid off brilliantly. I was confident that we were able to make critical adjustments in our life. Alzheimer's would require nothing less.

## CHAPTER 3

# Smelling Trouble

By 2001, when Phil was sixty-one years old, our happily anticipated retirement was becoming peculiar. In January our youngest child, Christopher, was home from college in Montana. He joined Phil and me for supper in the kitchen. A football playoff game was on TV. Our dogs were asleep in front of the fireplace. Relaxed and together, we were glad for a quiet evening, the busy holidays behind us. One of the commentators was talking about the Great One at Green Bay. "I know who that was," I chirped. Phil couldn't retrieve the name. Chris evidently didn't know. Lightheartedly I called out, "Vince Lombardi!" victoriously. Phil took offense.

He called me aside later and said I'd embarrassed him in front of Chris. He said that he felt personally exposed and that I was to blame. I was stunned. My immediate reaction was "Don't be ridiculous!" But his expression and accusing eyes stopped me. Instead, I apologized: "Please know that I'd never intentionally try to make you look stupid in front of anyone." My apology was not accepted; he fumed. I was mad by then, too, but I let it go.

The next day I recalled the Lombardi incident to Chris. He hadn't registered either my zealousness or his dad's silent response. I didn't tell Phil that I'd gone back to Chris because I didn't want to escalate the matter or make him feel worse. I just needed a reality check.

Chris returned to school. Phil and I packed for our winter stay in Texas. After the long road trip, we arrived tired. I fell into bed only to be

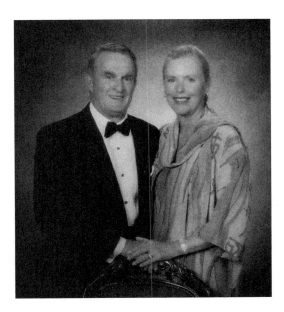

*Phil and me on a cruise in 2000*

met by a powerful dream that woke me up. Two vivid details lingered. One was dog smell, the other a stalled car engine. Wide awake, I got out of bed and went to the den to puzzle out the dream's meaning in my journal. I usually experienced sleep as a healthy escape from earthly matters—my dreams would quickly slip away with morning light. Not this time.

I wrote, "It's possible to live with dog smell until one no longer smells it." I didn't want to do that! As for a car engine, I had little interest in how it worked, but I'd always counted on it doing so. These images seemed important in my present circumstance. Basically something smelled, and I couldn't see why things were not working.

I admitted to myself that I was growing weary swimming in family crosscurrents. My folks were suffering the vagaries of old age in Florida. Our adult children and grandchildren were spread across the continent. These other generations welcomed me into and excused me from their lives, calling only intermittently on my love and wisdom. They all had other sustaining relationships.

I was most worried about my well-being in the context of Phil's well-being, and his in the context of mine. He seemed to count on me exclusively. He was uncomfortable with intermittency, now wanting to do everything together. I felt stranded with him on a desert island in the middle of Texas Hill Country.

In April I flew home to help Heidi as she was about to deliver her fourth child. When I called Phil with the good news of Susan's birth, he demanded grumpily, "Are you coming back or not?"

Our long planned trip to Norway with Phil's sister Allie and her husband, Rich, gave us a July break from our exclusive togetherness. We left Bergen on a coastal steamer to travel north and explore fjords. When we tied up in small ports along the way, Phil would take the shore map and set off enthusiastically for the city center. We would arrive at a point of interest having taken an indirect path. We family travelers accepted the confusion and misdirection as a kind of joke. I was not amused, however, when Phil kept landing his piece on the wrong point in our game of backgammon. I thought he was trying to rattle me on purpose and calmly insisted he redo his plays. Rich was observing us and asked me afterwards, "What was going on? Allie would have a fit if I played like that." In private I asked Phil about it. He admitted he couldn't concentrate.

That fall Phil and I set out on our own boat trip on the St. Croix River. Family visitors in August had left us happily exhausted. We were both anxious for some private, rejuvenating time on the river. Dressed in sweaters for the crisp breeze, we boarded with lots of provisions and high hopes. Phil took the helm. It was midweek, and no other boats were about. We had the river to ourselves.

The channel markers leaving home port were familiar, but Phil ignored them. Alarmed, I warned, "Phil, it's too shallow outside the channel." He waved off my caution. In no time a loud grinding noise and lurch brought us both to attention. We had not just run aground; we had caught the underwater wing dam that helped keep the channel open. We backed off, but our steering had become unreliable. We limped back to the service dock to have the damage assessed. Staff pulled the boat. One shaft and both propellers needed to be replaced.

This costly mistake was not from lack of experience or bad weather; it was plain poor judgment.

What was going on? How could I make sense of it? Who could help us? Back at the house Phil wept in my arms. We agreed to see a counselor together, someone who had helped a newly retired couple we knew. I made the appointment.

Prior to the first meeting, I wrote a lengthy letter to the psychologist giving some background information. I showed the letter to Phil, who approved my sending it after a cursory reading. I determined to remain relatively quiet in the first session, so he could express himself. Counseling was not his natural platform. As a surgeon, he was more inclined to cut out a problem and move on.

In the letter I confessed that I didn't always claim the private time I needed. I felt guilty leaving Phil for too long or too often. I didn't know how to help him. I wanted to understand and support him, and at the same time I also needed understanding and support. I admitted we were both tired, telling her, "When Phil sags, I sag too."

To reveal Phil's personality and frustration I contrasted two recent events for her. On a happy day he spent hours organizing his hunting and fishing gear and loading the car to the brim for the following morning's departure. Heidi and her young sons stopped by and ended up helping Grandpa catch grasshoppers for bait. Shrieks of delight ensued. On a crabby day Phil insisted on going to the bank in town *immediately* to ask a question that could have been handled on the phone. Instead we arrived unexpectedly, with Phil's confusing questions causing staff to scramble ineffectively to satisfy their important customer, Dr. Roy. I couldn't turn him off or straighten out the message. He groused at everyone else's incompetence.

Once in the counseling session, Phil talked about forgetting members' names at the golf club and forgetting his pitching wedge by the green. He admitted to feeling peripheral in some of the family goings-on. By our third session, the therapist recommended a psychiatrist for further consultation and possible medication for depression.

Phil was anxious that no one except me know he was seeking help. The idea that he might actually be helped was a great relief to me. I was anguished, not knowing what to do for him, what to say, what to confront, what to ignore, what was real, and what was a figment of my imagination.

Prescription depression medication helped ease Phil's darkened outlook and, in turn, lightened my despair. When we finally arrived in Florida in November, he was delighted with our new winter home. His sunnier disposition and embedded charm made it easy for him to make new friends on the golf course. He was as glad to take supper to my folks as I was to make it. Moving our winter residence had been a good decision, and 2002 was a sweet year for us.

By the spring of 2003 things were offtrack again. Phil admitted that he could not calculate the golf handicaps when he played with other men. When we took my folks out to dinner for Mother's birthday, I happened to notice that he'd written down a $400 tip. "Oh, Phil, the lighting is bad in here. May I help you?" I said, which allowed me to make a quick correction. On the drive home to Minnesota from Florida, his driving was fine, but his map reading was worthless. I was very worried about him. We made plans to go together to the Mayo Clinic for full physicals.

In late May I left Phil for the day to go to a fundraising conference in Minneapolis. In the middle of a session, I was handed a message that my husband had had an accident, and I was to meet my daughter Heidi in the emergency room at Woodwinds Hospital. The thirty-minute drive felt like hours. I was so relieved to see Phil and to be at his side.

He was lying on the table in the emergency room, with his unshaven face etched in pain and bewilderment. His old jeans had been cut from his frame; his dirty, misshapen Fleet Farm socks were still on. My discombobulated husband was in tatters, drained of authority and acutely broken.

At home alone, determined to remove some branches from a cedar tree by the house, Phil had selected several different types of ladders and saws from the garage. We will never know exactly what happened, but he, all of his equipment, and a few branches ended up on the ground. His pelvis was shattered.

I felt awful on so many fronts. Poor Phil was in agony if he moved. I had not been with him, paying attention. Luckily he had a portable house phone with him and managed to call Heidi's house. When the nanny picked up the message some time later, she called Heidi, who hurried to her dad's rescue. What if Heidi had not gotten the message? Phil had not thought to call 911; Heidi, herself a doctor, did. She also called her sister Jena in Boston and gave her the assignment of finding me.

Heidi observed Phil's unexpected confusion in a hospital setting. She tried to make him more comfortable. She brought him a CD player, magazines, and favorite treats. Suffering hospital delirium, Phil was terrified of invisible spiders coming out of the ceiling. I slept overnight in his room to hold his hand. The CT scan showed no sign of a concussion, but the doctor told me that Phil's brain was "small." I didn't understand. I knew that brain, small or not, was highly intelligent.

Our daughter Beth was in town from New York City on a consulting project with a large nonprofit. She was used to assembling data for good decision making and urged me, "Get Dad tested." I did. The results were unsettling. The neuropsychologist was not willing or perhaps not licensed to make a diagnosis, but he showed me Phil's bizarre responses. Phil did not correctly correlate objects. Shown a spoon, a hairbrush, and a comb, he did not put the hairbrush and comb together. Attempting to replicate a geometric drawing, he had drawn a picture of a lake and trees that he had narrated with a story to explain where the road went.

The doctors extended Phil's stay in the hospital, assigning him to the traumatic brain injury unit. Following instructions was hard for Phil. The success of his pelvic surgery depended on his compliance in rehabilitation. I pushed his wheelchair to those daily sessions and learned the restrictions for his movement.

I parroted the litany of instructions: "Put your right foot forward, slide your hips to the edge of the chair, push up on the chair arms to stand on the left leg, take the walker for balance. . . ." At home I had a ramp built to our front door so that Phil could finally escape the hospital after nearly a month.

Together we continued to work on his physical recovery. I was the safety officer. Phil was not supposed to lift objects or step on his right leg. He needed encouragement *and* supervision—like a young child. That he was an adult with a lot of independent-living experience compounded the difficult situation of his being housebound. Pain provided no caution; he no longer hurt. My job was to ensure that his bones were not jarred or bumped.

We did leave the house to go to the hospital for a prescribed MRI of his head. The result was "normal" for a sixty-three-year-old man. There was no evidence of stroke and no explanation of his thinking skips. The doctors told me Phil's confusion might lift suddenly, or incrementally, or not at all.

Our temporary suspension of activities while his bones mended was less daunting than the prospect of permanent scrambled thinking. That worry was the proverbial stone in my shoe, pushing into my tender sole. In occupational therapy sessions Phil refused to practice the money-counting exercise. He could not complete elementary mazes. I had told the doctors about Phil's thinking problems before the accident. They could not tell me if these glaring cognitive issues showing up now were related to Phil's traumatic fall or to a prior condition.

On Phil's July 9 birthday I declared a time-out for good behavior. Avoiding rush-hour traffic, I drove us carefully to Minneapolis for a 2:45 p.m. showing of *Winged Migration* and an early dinner out. We set aside the wine list. Phil sipped coffee before the meal instead. AWOL, we toasted ourselves with our water glasses. "Thank you, Barbara," Phil smiled appreciatively. "I love you, Philly," I responded. Clink!

By August Phil was pretty agile on crutches. I couldn't tell how much weight he was bearing on his right leg. The doctors were now allowing thirty to forty pounds of pressure. I only offered caution when he would set off *without* his crutches. As usual, Phil often didn't wait or think before he struck out, and he seemed to be more impulsive than ever. I was exhausted watching and trying to let go of him simultaneously.

On August 30 our daughter Beth married a Canadian man, Oliver, who worked with her at the consulting firm. To accommodate Phil, they thoughtfully designed an intimate wedding with only family members to be conducted on Heidi's deck overlooking the St. Croix River, and they made sure I had no responsibility for any of the planning.

Our oldest daughter, Jena, flew from her home in Boston to Florida to collect my mother. My brother, Ted, flew to Florida to care for my frail father so that Mother could leave. Chris flew in from the West, Oliver's family flew in from Toronto, and his uncle from the United Kingdom. Seeing Phil look so much like himself before the wedding was reassuring to all.

Dressing for the ceremony, Phil became slightly agitated tying his tie. His cursing reminded me of my own father in frustration. The knot Phil finally achieved had the seam on the tie's back showing in the loop of the knot. In the scheme of things it was definitely unimportant.

Arriving at the ceremony, Phil left his crutches in the car and insisted on walking down forty steps unassisted to the deck. He was excited, noncompliant, and inconsiderate. The many months I'd been working with him on his recovery regime were discarded. In my momentary exasperation, I told our son, Chris, "If your dad falls, call 911 and ride with him to the hospital." Phil did not fall. His happiness to be there kept him upright. We celebrated the sacred moment as one family. The experience was a potent reminder to me of what was most important.

As Phil and I lay close together in early morning light, I told him I knew that this period of our life was for family—us, my folks, the children, the grandchildren. I also knew it was time to resign from the Wilder Foundation board of directors, which I had served for thirteen years. When we got up, I immediately went to my desk and wrote my letter of resignation. Setting aside this valued connection was a huge concession for me but the right thing to do. My life had been so abundant. Wilder's commitment to helping vulnerable folks toward a better life was dear to me. When I called the board chair to say directly how much Wilder's mission meant, I burst into tears. Then I mailed the letter that day. Without fully understanding why or how, I knew Phil needed me in new ways.

# CHAPTER 4

△▽▽▽△

# Getting Help

Admitting any personal problem was hard for Phil. His unwillingness to face his own vulnerability I attributed to his type A personality, his surgeon's need to be in charge, some manly necessity to be strong, his general lack of self-awareness, his difficulty in asking for help, plain stubbornness, fear, denial, or almost anything but the fact he was incapable of understanding his own medical problem.

His release from Hennepin County Medical Center in June 2003 stated that he was to see a neurologist. He did not disrespect the specialty, but I remembered during his internship how he hated that rotation. "Watering the vegetables," he called it. To him such patient care had been too unhopeful and incremental. I wondered how he felt now that he needed neurological services himself. I tried to be hopeful. I was definitely eager for any incremental improvement he might make.

The neurologist rounding at HCMC with students did not impress me. He made no attempt to engage Phil or acknowledge me as his wife. He swooped into Phil's room, presented Phil as a specimen, told the students that Phil had shown great confusion possibly associated with Alzheimer's, and led the contingent back into the hall.

Our meeting with a neurologist in St. Paul was friendly and gracious. Dr. Ormiston knew Phil as Phil. He spent time examining him and chatting with both of us. He tried to reassure Phil that even though his symptoms showed some kind of early dementing illness, he would not face any imminent or precipitous slide. He wrote a prescription for

Aricept and gave me a copy of *The 36-Hour Day*. In the car Phil told me not to worry. "I can't get Alzheimer's until I'm at least seventy." He was sixty-three. He did not comprehend his sentence. I told him not to worry and promised, "We'll be a team." Inside I vacillated between defensive disbelief and urgency to know more.

On medication Phil did not seem to improve or get any worse mentally. He was mostly interested in his pelvic fracture healing and ridding himself of his physical restrictions. When we returned to the orthopedic office in November 2003, the X-rays showed that Phil's bones had slipped and that he needed a hip replacement. I was sick, mad, and scared. The thought of Phil enduring another surgery, spiders reappearing to him, and more rehab was unbearable. All my efforts to help him be compliant seemed for naught. How much more could either of us take? The orthopedist showed us a suitcase full of hip joints and recommended the type that could be glued into place for immediate strength. The day of the surgery I slumped in the waiting room, resigned that I would be resuming my job of chief safety officer.

These worries were misplaced. The surgical outcome was excellent. Phil was discharged pain-free within forty-eight hours. The familiar rehab routine with his ready use of crutches was no problem. Grateful for the skilled care, I was even more proud of Phil's grit.

I reminded myself to calm down. My anxiety served no one and made me tired. It wasn't the kind of tired that sleep necessarily remedied. My effort to take care of myself was becoming a weird combination of self-imposed calm and frantic urges to hurry up about it. With Heidi's encouragement, I went to the gym to learn strengthening exercises. The first session left me lame. Then I caught a nasty cold.

In December Phil was walking well and eager to join holiday festivities. At granddaughter Jane's school concert he chatted happily with people he did not know, giving them lengthy explanations of his recent hip surgery. When he put his arm up the sleeve of one unsuspecting woman to demonstrate how the surgery was performed, Heidi gently steered him away.

Before the end of the year, we had to fill out a Social Security Administration questionnaire regarding his disability claim. Phil's effort and responses were tortured. He tried hard to focus but missed distinctions like "before" and "after." He repeated the same answer to different questions, skipping back and forth between questions and filling in any white space with random phrases. I sent a copy of the questionnaire to Phil's doctor, since the SSA would be contacting him. I felt as if I were sending in a rectal smear.

After the holidays we flew to our winter residence in Florida, leaving our medical community behind. Phil deserved to escape patient mode. I needed a dose of denial. Phil could play golf but not drive the car. His fractured pelvis had made driving impossible. With his thinking issues exposed, I didn't allow him to resume. Instead he operated the golf cart, following the cart path from our condo to the course inside the gated community. Independent of me, he played with the guys once a week. He also tended shelves of orchid plants on our porch. Life felt sort of normal.

Then one night in January, just as Phil and I were getting ready for bed, the phone rang. It was Mother. "Your father is screaming in pain. I've called an ambulance." I urged Phil to go to bed and jumped into the car. The ambulance was already there when I pulled up. Dad was moaning on the gurney just coming out the front door. In panicked anger and pain, he spit out, "What are you doing here?" Obviously unable to help him, I blurted out, "I've come to take care of Mother."

Fortunately Heidi and her two little girls were visiting my parents. Leaving the sleeping children with Mother, Heidi and I drove to the hospital so she could advocate for her grandfather. Heidi and the other doctors agreed to emergency abdominal surgery to repair a likely stomach perforation. I took Heidi back to the condo, found Dad's necessary papers, and brought Mom back to the surgery waiting room. We did not know if Dad would survive the surgery, but he did. Over the next few days Heidi interpreted the intensive care scene for Mother and me. My heart broke for Phil that no one was asking his advice, despite his thirty-five years of medical experience.

As Dad's surgical recovery progressed, Heidi left, and our oldest daughter and her two children, ages nine and ten, arrived from Boston to stay with Mother. Jena's loving support allowed us all to hold on. Mother had another trusted companion in residence. Phil had his big grandchildren to enjoy. And I had a soul mate in my daughter. She and I maintained a gentle flow of changing family combinations for hospital visits, pool time, and meals.

The level of extended family support could not last forever. Neither did Dad's recovery. Two days after Jena's team left, Mother and I faced a decision that I'm sure Dad had wanted us to make. We called my brother back from his honeymoon so he could say good-bye to Dad, and together we instituted hospice.

The next morning Phil and I went to see Dad at six. I excused the night nurse and took Dad's hand. The doctor came in briefly, pushed Dad's eyes open, and addressed him, "Edgar!" Deeply asleep, Dad did not respond. Looking at me, the doctor expressed concern for Mother and recommended that I try to keep her calm and see to her rest. He did not know of Phil's health issues. I clung to Dad's last words to me, "Barbara, sit down and stop fussing." I trusted that we would find our way forward. Dad died the next day.

Turning my attention to Dad in his waning days and then to Mother alone after seventy years of marriage, I tried not to think about Phil riding his bicycle unaccompanied. I felt he was safe in the golf cart on the obvious golf cart path, but biking neighborhood streets amid so many lookalike buildings was a different matter. If Phil got lost or fell, he would need help and have trouble asking for it.

Phil's compassion was in full force at Dad's passing, but he soon lost patience with Mom. He complained that he was invisible in her eyes— and he was right about that. All of our emotions were roiling. Good friends invited my brother, Mom, Phil, and me to a quiet supper at their home. Phil was tired. I held Mom's icy hand.

When Phil and I got back to our place, he was agitated. "Your Mother talks about our daughters as if they were hers. She never gives me any credit!" he fumed. I listened to him rant. My head pounded. Arguing with Phil's hypersensitivity would have been cruel and useless. I felt like a punching bag. We went to bed.

Awake in the middle of the night, I cried for Dad, made a silent promise to look after Mom, and worried about Phil. It was hard to take it all in or to let it out. "Breathe," I told myself.

Phil's and my journey with Alzheimer's lived in the family garden of both sorrow and joy. Our youngest daughter, Beth, soon arrived in Florida to partner with Mother. When Beth told Phil privately that she was expecting, he was thrilled. Happy news bucked us all up. She suggested I buy Phil a puppy. Phil loved dogs. I merely liked them. Having something else to care for did not immediately appeal to me, but I saw the kindness and wisdom in her idea. Phil had been trying so hard to make our life work. He'd been surviving on his abundant social skill, sense of humor, and athleticism on the golf course. A gift of puppy love was the perfect reward.

Phil missed his Brittany spaniel, Lily, back in Minnesota. Before my father died, a brown and white puppy had caught Phil's eye in a pet shop window. I had put him off: "How can we train a puppy when we're on the golf course so much?" Whenever we went to the movies, Phil wandered next door to peer in the pet shop window again. The small Cavalier King Charles pup was just the right size for our condo. With Beth's encouragement, we returned to the shop and signed purchase papers. We named the little guy Sunny for Florida sunshine.

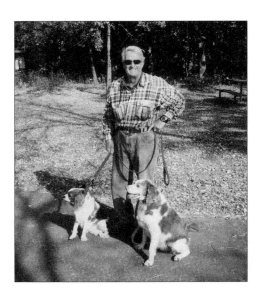

*Phil with Sunny and Lily*

Having a new dog gave Phil happy news to tell our friends, who did not yet know our secret of his dementing illness. The dog was an uncomplicated subject on which he could speak easily from his heart. I found great comfort in holding the warm bundle myself. Our new carpeting seemed unimportant.

Phil was in charge of Sunny's carrier on our May flight back to Minnesota. They were the best of pals. I was grateful for Phil's preoccupation, which allowed me space to dispense our luggage and find the right gate. Airline policy required Sunny to stay in the carrier. Phil could not follow that rule. Soon after the plane took off, Sunny was in Phil's lap. The stewardess reminded him pleasantly to put the dog back. I encouraged his cooperation too, but neither of us was successful for long. Phil retrieved Sunny over and over again. In the end, an airplane blanket loosely covered Phil's infraction. They slept, and I relaxed.

Back in Minnesota, we reconnected with all Phil's professional helpers again. For the first time, Dr. Ormiston used the diagnosis of Alzheimer's directly with Phil. Phil didn't want to wear a big A on his head and have everyone know. I knew it would not be a surprise to our loved ones. The doctor encouraged me to call our children. I told him that Phil and I had plans to celebrate our fortieth wedding anniversary by taking a trip to Alaska. I was sure we would enjoy it despite the challenges that Alzheimer's entailed. When I called Beth with the doctor's diagnosis, she used humor to digest the Alzheimer's message. "If you fall overboard when you're in Alaska, I'll fish you out. You don't get to swim with the bears. You are taking care of Dad!" We laughed.

Phil and I sailed out of Sitka aboard Lindblad's *Sea Lion*. The natural beauty of the area and the wildlife brightened our spirits. We kayaked in a salmon stream and hiked in a rain forest. We followed naturalists on birding expeditions. Flocks of mottled sandpipers burst from the sand flats at low tide. A single yellow-legged lesser sandpiper patrolled a small creek, warning loudly against our approach. Traveling in small motor boats called Zodiacs, we saw dozens of eagles, a lone swan, slender arctic terns, belted kingfishers, red-throated loons, marbled murrelet, and great blue herons. Safely aboard the *Sea Lion*, we watched a black bear on shore. Aiming our binoculars we could see its tan nose and prominent ears. These discoveries were plain fun.

I took a break from observing wildlife and joined a few passengers in a poetry/reflection time on the aft deck. A young park ranger led the exercise. We took ten minutes to compose haikus. I wrote two about a coyote:

> Lithe orange-stockinged legs
> On scent, tail out, ears up, go,
> Ship unnoticed, hunt.

> Shelled shore, bending grass
> Lone coyote, focused, circling…
> What is he up to?

It struck me as soon as I finished that the images were about Phil as well as the coyote. When we took turns to read, tears filled my eyes. I surprised myself by telling the small group that Phil had just been diagnosed with Alzheimer's.

When I returned to Phil, he had written to me on a ship's postcard. It was a list of misspelled animals interspersed with "hoorahs" and signed "Mr. Alzheimer's a.k.a. Roy Boy." We took refuge in being by ourselves for a while, watching the sea lions from our stateroom window.

Some days were very cold. Phil's layered clothing did not always include his warmest jacket. While we were watching for whales, the cold drove him inside. When I joined him in the salon, he and seven-year-old Danielle were giggling. She was drawing his portrait. She showed a cloud-like brain above his head and question marks in his cheeks. He was pleased with her rendering. Danielle joined us for Scrabble. Soon an adult guest, Joan, allied herself with Phil. Together they formed words and progressed the game. Without keeping score, we simply took turns until all the tiles were used. Phil unexpectedly confided his Alzheimer's diagnosis to Joan, only to learn that she was a committed volunteer for Faith in Action, which helps families who have a loved one suffering from dementia.

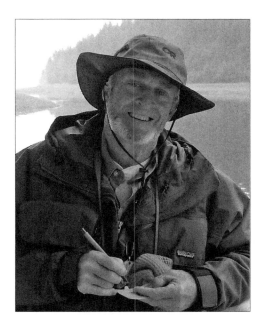

*Phil in Alaska, 2004*

Being with people who accepted us as we were was very reassuring. I was particularly encouraged by Phil's willingness to engage with other passengers and the naturalists. He asked one guide how to distinguish between sea lions and mountain lions. The fellow paused and respectfully said, "That's an interesting question."

I hoped the second week up to Denali would not be too much. The bumpy bus ride into the park frustrated Phil, who was trying to use his binoculars, but the flight around Denali and the hike up Blueberry Hill pleased him. We wore our bug suits to ward off the mosquitoes. He liked having the right equipment. As we walked along, he sincerely thanked me for going on the trip with him. He wanted a souvenir of the expedition and decided a rock would be perfect. He found a brick-sized piece of mica that I encouraged him to put back. "Phil, consider yourself a window shopper," I told him. "Let's just look. We don't need to keep anything." Moments later he found a smaller igneous rock with an intrusion of quartz and slipped it into his backpack. Some things would never change.

At dinner we sat next to a woman who was beginning to get on Phil's nerves. She was an experienced hiker, a wilderness writer, a spirited conversationalist, and a large presence. Phil's lighthearted one-liners were no match. On the trip out of the park he was determined to stay clear of her. At the airport the next morning she gave him a big farewell hug and told me she thought we were very lucky in our relationship.

Phil had ended up telling everyone he was on medication for Alzheimer's. The trip had been a good chance to practice being upfront. We were not cast out like lepers of old. We were still ourselves, Barbara and Phil.

Back at home we watched devastating Florida hurricane reports on the evening news and thought about our friends there. I suggested to Phil that we send them a letter that revealed his Alzheimer's diagnosis. He was no longer worried about wearing a big A on his head and approved my idea. On October 8, 2004, I wrote the following letter:

> We certainly hope that you've weathered hurricane season and that it is over. It's hard to imagine the power that caused so much property damage and psychological wear.
>
> Phil and I find ourselves blowing in a very different kind of wind. While neither surprised nor totally flattened, we are adjusting to Phil's recent diagnosis of Alzheimer's. Our appreciation for life and our senses of humor continue to sustain us as we journey forward. The idea is to live in the moment. When we get it right, life delights us. When we fall back to old ways of over planning and piling up commitments, life sometimes trips us up. The doctors suggest simplifying our life; practical reality shows us that simple can be elusive. Still, we are most grateful to know the Good in life.
>
> We are having fun. Our recent 40th wedding anniversary trip to Alaska filled us with natural wonder and happy companionship. Our golf outings continue to amuse us. Phil shot his first hole in one, witnessed by his hunting buddies, who are used to his old shotgun accuracy. And, many days we are in our meadow, planting yet more wild flowers with our Florida puppy in tow. Phil has affectionately renamed little Sunny Einstein.

Our Minnesota friends remind us with deep affection that we are all dealing with some health issue or another. While the issues challenge us to live in new ways, they do not define us. We are looking forward to seeing you as we are. Just when we will get to Florida and how long we will stay, however, are unscheduled at the moment. Come winter we will likely want to trade our snow shovels for golf clubs.

We'll stay in touch.

Dr. Ormiston also set up an appointment at the Mayo Clinic for a second opinion. The full checkup confirmed Phil's plight. The vague hope that some other—curable—problem was at play did not materialize. Phil managed the oral questions with equanimity, mostly because he had no sense of his own inaccuracy. He didn't know George Washington was the first president. He was happy and confident with his answer of John Adams. The written testing brought tears to his eyes. Watching him struggle crushed me as well. Trying to make something positive of the appointment, we offered to be part of any appropriate trials. Nothing fit. I bought *Mayo Clinic on Alzheimer's Disease* for future reference. We left deflated.

Dr. Ormiston referred us on to Bethesda Rehabilitative Hospital in St. Paul to see Dr. Holm, who specialized in dementia care. Bethesda had previously been a full-service hospital where Phil had performed surgery and helped to train family medicine residents. Going there to see Dr. Holm was like going home. Phil knew the much younger Dr. Holm, though he'd never worked with him directly. We both trusted this new man—Phil because he knew him, and me because I wanted a dementia specialist on our team.

Dr. Holm took great care of us in the office and welcomed my intervening phone calls and questions. He couldn't make Phil better in the long run, but he observed Phil knowingly, accepted my honest reporting, and managed the medications that Phil was taking to stabilize his mood and improve his concentration.

Dr. Holm represented excellence in a medical model of care. He was very knowledgeable about the disease and very skilled in caring for his patients. But he only saw Phil quarterly for an hour. The rest of the days and weeks and months, Phil was in my care.

Phil obsessed about Lily and Sunny. We took them for walks twice a day. He dressed them in multiple collars and bought lots of bright colored leashes. He could not *not* feed them scraps during dinner. They swarmed under the table like sharks at the fish cleaning station. I picked my battles very carefully in our peculiar circumstance and reluctantly gave the dogs a lot of slack. I gently noted, "Phil, you're spoiling the dogs. They shouldn't overeat." He'd smile and soon slip them another bit of his dinner.

When Lily died, Phil worried incessantly that Sunny needed a buddy. Reasoning with him or trying to change his Alzheimer's mind was impossible. Our good friends' son showed Cavalier King Charles dogs. He generously gave us Mariah, a beautiful retired champion. In high style, she pranced on her leash and barked if Sunny got in front of her. Sunny pulled as if he were trying out for the Iditarod and naturally got ahead of her on our walks. "Whoa, Sunny," Phil commanded. I tried to urge Mariah forward. Then we would switch. Phil and Mariah would lead, while I nearly strangled poor Sunny in restraint. My solution was an Invisible Fence and their running free.

The installers marked the fence line with occasional white flags for our reference. A trainer came to teach us and the dogs how to use the fence. Phil did not like the woman handling his dogs. He was rude. She cut our lesson short, offering "good luck" to me. The dogs soon learned their limits, but Phil did not. As if by magnetic attraction, he proceeded to plant or dig up something where the underground wire ran. An alarm would sound in the garage. I would have to turn off the power, apply an electrical patch, and reset the system. Keeping track of the dogs, Phil, and the new system was a crazy-making job.

One day Heidi called to ask me to watch her little girls while she picked up her sons from elementary school. I told Phil, "I'll be home in less than an hour." When I returned, the dogs greeted the car, but Phil was nowhere in sight. I set out on foot to find him. He was not in our meadow. I walked down to the river and around the neighbors' houses, calling his name. Nothing. I got back in the car, searching local streets for an hour in a panic. Finally he came into view. He could see I was upset. "I've been looking for Sunny," he explained, oblivious to the idea that he himself had been missing.

In early 2005 I heard about a support group at the University of Minnesota that offered a family-centered model of care. The idea of Phil and me attending a support group with strangers was a stretch—both of us liked our privacy—but I was desperate for more help.

I told Phil that we might be able to "help with a project" at the university. He was proud of his affiliation with the University of Minnesota Medical School. I made an appointment for us to find out more. Actually, it was an interview with the Family Caregiving Center leader, who would decide if we were the right candidates to join his support group. Wayne Caron was a compassionate genius in understanding family dynamics with dementing illness in the mix. Rumpled, funny, and totally nonthreatening, he embraced Phil's personhood. Phil told Wayne all about himself and us. Wayne told Phil that we'd be a big help if we joined the group he was working with. Phil left with the good feeling of being of service. I was glad we had a new weekly activity we could do together.

Each Saturday morning, Wayne lectured the first hour to the whole group on a range of topics aimed at honoring the person with memory loss, not fixing the disease. His recurring messages that a person did not lose capacity until it was gone and that capacity could be nurtured were reassuring. He cited research and showed bullet-point slides in an academic approach that suited Phil's background. Support group members interrupted freely to ask questions or offer observations. I really appreciated Wayne's positive outlook and took notes.

The second hour he separated the family caregivers into a different room. We had a chance to tell our stories to each other and gain strength from others' firsthand experiences. The first Saturday I listened deeply to other family members who were further along the Alzheimer's journey than Phil and I were. One woman described the time she was expecting someone to drive her husband home from a meeting, but her husband never showed up. After many phone calls, a car trip to the meeting place, and two hours of worry, the police called to ask her to

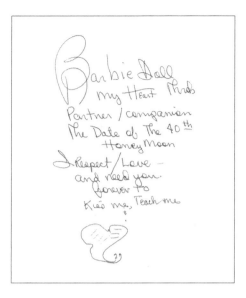

*A note from Phil to me, June 2004*

pick up her husband at a convenience store. He'd tried to walk home, become disoriented, and fortunately made himself understood by the officer, who just happened to stop at the convenience store. Her honest reporting showed both her husband's vulnerability and her own loving endurance. Seeing our predicament played out by others gave me courage to carry on. Knowing I wasn't the only one trying to keep life together helped somehow.

Thus armed with weekly family-centered care meetings and an accessible, competent dementia physician, Phil and I lived into his diagnosis. Phil's odd, eruptive, changeable behavior had a name: Alzheimer's. I knew he was doing the best he could. I tried to do my best to keep him in his comfort zone where he could still be Phil.

# CHAPTER 5

# Maintaining Friendships

Despite professional guidance, our circumstance was naturally scary. Our sixties were supposed to be our golden years, having completed our commitments to work and raising children. Like our longtime friends, we wanted to believe in the modern fairy tale of a robust retirement, when grandchildren, recreation, adventure, and new learning lay ahead. Learning about Alzheimer's was not what we had in mind. Knowing that the chances of getting the disease were related to age was enough to tuck away. We didn't feel old. To ourselves, we didn't even look that old.

I easily overlooked Phil's subtle Alzheimer's-related behaviors, which our friends often accepted as quirks. As much as I sensed something was the matter as early as 2001, I was not looking for trouble. To the contrary, I was busy filling up our new retirement with plans. Building a small house in our Minnesota meadow and switching our winter residence from Texas to Florida were meant to simplify our lives. Planning was my forte.

By 2003, Phil's and my partnership had become a full-time job for me in which I tried to preserve a sense of ordinary living. He needed my companionship to participate successfully. At the same time I had to give him some space. Being outside was the best way to do that. Working in the yard was ideal. I enjoyed deadheading the echinacea and scattering the seed. The task was endless and pleasurable. I liked to smell the earth and feel the sun on my shoulders. Phil smiled at me from a distance, enjoying his own effort and satisfied that we were both "working" together.

Cleaning the garage was another joint endeavor that went fairly well. I turned to that activity repeatedly as the weather grew colder. Discarding unnecessary stuff and discovering old treasures entertained Phil. A spray can of florescent orange paint particularly pleased him. He sprayed the chain-link dog-kennel fence, which I didn't really care about. When he slipped out of view briefly and also covered our new mailbox, I was not happy with the unsightly mess. Somehow I managed to institute a rule that the paint can had to stay in the garage, that it could not come in the house.

Going into town to the home of our friends Sandy and Bruce Kiernat for supper, I did not notice that Phil had slipped the can into his jacket pocket before getting into the car. When Sandy greeted us at the door, she immediately eyed the can with alarm. Inside I caught on to the situation. Offhandedly and calmly, I said, "Oh, Phil, that can has to stay outside." He relinquished it, and I put it on the front porch until departure. Fortunately, we didn't test the depth of our friendship with an unsolicited redecorating of their lovely foyer.

The garage also produced a snow blower that interested Phil with winter approaching. He could not get it started, so we took it to a small-engine shop. It was accepted at delivery, but we got a call later refusing the work. The shop owner no longer wanted to deal with Phil; he remembered being stiffed on a previous chipper repair. Phil's position was that the repair was never completed properly. At the time I had been glad that the piece of equipment was sidelined. Now I was frustrated, seeing both sides.

In the end, Phil was willing for me to call back to sort out the problem. He monitored the call, scrutinizing my explanation and plea for service without revealing his "mix-ups." After we picked up the repaired blower, Phil could not find the handle he'd removed so the unit would fit in the car. All the consternation and effort finally netted a working machine that allowed Phil to run through the first light snowfall with a real sense of accomplishment. I felt as if I'd plowed a drift with a spatula.

Heidi's family invited us on their 2004 Thanksgiving trip to New Mexico for a break. The mountain snow would not be our responsibility, and I could relax into a broader set of loving relationships. Phil and seven-year-old grandson Tommy had a fit of giggles at dinner one night. Phil enjoyed walking the family dog. I swam with the children. We all hiked before supper and enjoyed magnificent sunsets. Our struggles seemed smaller in the larger landscape.

When we returned home, a social worker from the human service agency Family Means came to our home to interview Phil and me about our need for respite care. Bruce Kiernat had volunteered to take respite training from the agency so he could help us out. Initially Phil was too busy to talk with the worker. He had important work to do in the garage. "Come in when you can," I called to him and then used the time to ask questions of my own. When Phil joined us in the kitchen, he was polite but didn't stay long. Talking about his friend Bruce to the social worker, he was not only coherent but full of affection and respect. Excusing himself, he lingered at the kitchen pass-through listening to what I might reveal. While he trusted me, he wanted to know what I was saying. Talking about him in his presence felt awkward at best. I chose my words carefully. How I said something mattered and required careful consideration.

The next week the Kiernats and the Roys and the social worker all met together and formally agreed to the helping arrangement. Bruce was newly retired. Phil thought that he would be helping his friend. Afterwards, we couples went to Perkins for the $3.99 senior breakfast special. Our easy togetherness was like old times. Bruce clapped Phil on the shoulder and thanked him, "You are a really good friend, Phil."

Christmas was soon upon us, and Jena invited us to spend the holiday with them in Boston. Phil and I were clearly slipping beyond the place of family leaders to one of respected elders with our children actively caring for our well-being. Jena did give us jobs, however. I grocery-shopped, prepared spinach salad, and mashed potatoes. Phil went with Jena to serve holiday treats in the grandchildren's classrooms. We all attended the Christmas Eve children's pageant. Max (age ten) was a talking shepherd, and Mimi (age nine) was a last-minute substitute wise man. At supper afterwards, Phil kept interrupting others with his appreciative remarks about the show.

Jena, her husband, and I returned to church for the midnight service. Our son, Chris, kept watch as the kids and grandpa slept. I sat alone while Jena and Marc helped serve communion. Blessings and memories of Christmases past flooded me. The reality of being on my own in the future hit me. Imagining other Christmas Eves without Phil stabbed my heart. My happy elf and companion would not sing "Silent Night" with me and welcome the midnight tolling of bells. Finding Jena at the back of the church following the service, I could not speak; my eyes filled with tears. Words failed. She embraced me and left Marc to collect the communion cups from the pews.

Max set the tone for Christmas morning. He had taken church candles, tied yellow ribbons around them, and wrapped them for a first gift of the day. He announced, "I have something for each of you." And then he explained, "The yellow ribbon is to remind us of our troops in Iraq, and the candle is to wish for peace." Tuning to his loving gift and the prospect of peace reset my heart in the moment. How fortunate our family was to be together!

Phil and I concluded the year of 2004 with dinner at the home of our dear friends Abby and Ken Dawkin. The evening's good feelings were another godsend. Phil talked to Ken about his idea to sell our Florida condo, he spoke openly about his Alzheimer's, and he relaxed into the comfort of old friendship and a quiet evening. We four enjoyed each other's stories of the holidays. As always, Abby's meal was delicious. The tempo of the evening was perfect. Phil sustained his attention. We even spent time reseated in the living room after supper. Abby would not allow the mood to be broken with group cleanup. When Phil said he was ready to go, we all supported the timing of the evening's conclusion. I was thankful not only for the time together but also for the promise of enduring friendship. Loving family and cherished friends would assuredly support us in the new year and days ahead.

In early 2005 Bruce Kiernat began the practice of multiple weekly outings with Phil. I was thrilled with possibilities of uninterrupted desk time and seeing my women friends again. My reluctance to sell the Florida condo, born mostly of the effort involved, melted away.

Receiving business calls at a time when I could talk easily was a hit-or-miss proposition, however. Phil complained bitterly that I excluded him from one call. Even though I knew to let the bile roll off my hide, I hated the insult. In confronting his agitated Alzheimer's mind, I had no appropriate defense or offense or diversion. The venting itself seemed to help him in the end. He had no understanding or patience for all the steps in a realty transaction.

Home with us for a few days, Chris watched us with a tender heart. He managed to spirit Phil away to play virtual golf one afternoon, so I could get a haircut. Our dinner table conversations were largely orations by Phil. Chris looked puzzled in trying to respond or enter into the word stream. I tried to assure him that Phil and I would do fine, that our life was just different. He occasionally gave me a shoulder hug and often a smile, which meant a lot. Then he went back to Montana.

Soon outings with Bruce fell apart. One day a series of errands concluding at Home Depot resulted in Bruce having to say no to Phil's insistence on purchasing a large piece of carpeting for the garage. Knowing that it was unneeded at our house, Bruce stressed to Phil that the carpet roll would not fit in the car. Having lost spatial understanding and not liking restrictions, Phil grew angry. Being told no really frosted him. When they returned home, Phil stomped into the house and declared that he would never speak to Bruce again. "Get out of here," he yelled.

Bruce looked apologetically at me and shrugged his shoulders. His words to smooth the day's closure were to no avail. I looked at Bruce knowingly and bid him farewell.

"Phil, what happened?" I asked. "He doesn't listen!" Phil replied. "He drags me around. There were so many bridges and trucks and stops." I settled him at the kitchen table and accepted his tirade. I was genuinely sorry that their easy fellowship had broken down. Phil could not let go of his vitriolic reaction to the restrictions Bruce had applied. He admitted that he'd never felt so angry toward someone he cared about. He did not want to go out with Bruce anymore! It was a chilling reminder to me that I was the primary caregiver.

On Sunday we went to church, where the pulpit flowers honored the one-year anniversary of Dad's death. Phil gladly told friends that we were selling our Florida condo. "I'd really only gone to Florida to look after Barbara's parents," he told them. I felt as if a wave was washing away the good friends and happy times we'd had there. After we got home and ate lunch, I needed to be alone. My mood was falling into despair. I felt the world closing in on me like the shrink-wrap that was used to cover our former boat for the winter. When I eventually went to see what Phil was up to, he'd found four battery chargers in the garage. He insisted that one could charge another. When I suggested otherwise, sparks flew literally and figuratively. The idea of a fire and our personal safety in jeopardy sunk me another notch.

On Monday I announced I had things to do. I excluded Phil from my business calls and desk work, partly to show him that being with me wasn't always such a good deal. Maybe he would rethink the appeal of outings with Bruce. When I intercepted him in the kitchen later, he was writing a donation check to public television. I reminded him that we had made a gift at year-end. He wanted to do more. "How much?" I asked. "Thirty dollars," he said firmly. He'd written the figure as $3,000 with no decimal point. The return envelope in hand was for public radio. I offered to get the correct address. Disregarding the payee on his check and looking at his preprinted envelope, he told me sternly, "MPR comes out of my radio." It was so hard for us to communicate!

The next week Bruce orchestrated a scaled-down outing that involved a trip to an orchid greenhouse and lunch. Phil accepted the invitation. They returned with beautiful specimens as Valentine gifts for Sandy and me. They were very pleased with themselves. Phil had allowed Bruce to check his sales slip and credit card receipt. I was as glad for their restored trust as for the plants. Trusted friendship erased any obvious sense of Phil's need for a caregiver. He could be his enthusiastic self. Seeing his happiness was a boost for me.

Spring came early in 2005. Sunshine and warmth drew us outside. We worked day after day cleaning out the flower beds around the house. Content being alone together and spent from physical effort, we were spiritually reenergized.

We were enthused to begin the golf season. Ken Dawkins and other fellows at the club took turns partnering with Phil on Friday mornings. Phil gladly left the score keeping to others. In fact, unbeknownst to him, he and his partner of the day were basically eliminated from the competition, as his memory of the rules was scant. Thankfully, compassionate camaraderie remained in full force. The invisible help of these friends buoyed Phil's spirits and gave me a new, weekly, four-hour respite for the summer!

The Dawkins, Kiernats, and other friends reached out to us over and over again. Accepting so much help was not exactly easy, though my gratitude was real. I had no time or way to repay all the kindnesses.

When asked, "How might I help you?" I often did not know what to ask for. Nothing could make Alzheimer's go away. In dealing with it, Phil had all the professional and family attention anyone could hope for. Friends tried to show him a good time. What did I need for myself? To relax and to laugh with a good friend.

These brief respites orchestrated by Bruce and Ken and others were critical in restoring my energy. Freedom from caregiving was essential in order to resume the job that was never done. These gifts of time away from Phil were a chance for me to stay connected to others: to hear their stories and to tell mine. I wanted to stay engaged in a world beyond Alzheimer's. Tending cherished friendships necessitated some independence from Phil. I never wanted to abandon him, but neither did I want to withdraw from life.

# CHAPTER 6

# Breaking Away

An introvert, I required private time to refuel. Phil's increasing dementia meant I had less and less of it. Arranging any separation was hard work even though our family and friends willingly replaced me in spending quality time with Phil. I wanted us to be together, but I also needed occasional time-outs. In 2004 and 2005, he was still full of life and the desire to enjoy it, and he resented any evidence of his lack of independence.

He naturally missed driving, which surfaced from time to time in angst or rage. "I don't want to wait around the golf club until you can come and get me," he seethed. I told him smoothly, "I'll be practicing putting while you are having lunch. We'll just go home together." Practicing putting was certainly no hardship, but it was not necessarily how I wanted to spend my limited free time. Occasionally one of the other golfers went out of his way to bring Phil home. Phil didn't really understand the inconvenience of our living out in the country forty minutes away from the club.

When he would demand to drive again, I would tell him evenly, "Phil, it's easy for me to take you anywhere whenever you want. You gave your license up, and I cancelled your insurance. We're saving money now." Sometimes he accepted the explanation. At other times he was determined to retake his driver's test and get his license back. We did stop at a license bureau to pick up the Minnesota State Driving Manual. I wasn't sure how much of the text he could comprehend.

He pestered me to the point that I made a bargain with him. I said I would make an appointment at the Courage Center, where a specialist could assess his readiness for driving. I was sure that their written and behind-the-wheel tests would reveal his incapacity in an objective way and that their experience in these matters would make their response both humane and final.

Radiating enthusiasm and friendliness, Phil happily climbed into the driver's seat of their training car. The evaluator later returned with Phil and, to my horror, said, "I only had to use the hand brake a couple of times. Phil would probably be safe in your neighborhood as long as you are in the car with him for prompts." What? I didn't have a hand brake in our car. And once in the driver's seat, Phil could go wherever he chose regardless of what I said. I put my foot down. "Phil, if we are both in the car, I will do the driving." My nerves could not stand coaching him at every turn and enforcing limits by the mile. Sadly for him, he never was able to make an appointment on his own to take the real driving test. He could not use the telephone book to find the phone number. I wouldn't help him in that process, but I did take extra care to make my chauffeuring seem effortless. I dreaded his occasional plea to drive, but I was tough. I knew he wasn't safe!

I'd become the family driver when Phil shattered his pelvis back in 2003 and stayed in the driver's seat thereafter. I didn't really mind. Being an independent medical wife and a country woman, I was used to being behind the wheel. Phil no longer opened the car door for me, but that was a small matter. Driving him places he wanted to go was not really a chore. In fact, as time went on, it was a valued activity that we could do together.

If I went out by myself in the car, however, Phil was essentially stranded. Only rarely and briefly did I leave him by himself after his confirmed diagnosis in 2004. The major exceptions and challenges were the births of our two granddaughters in New York City, one that fall and another in 2005.

First-born Caitlyn made her entry into the world on schedule. Beth didn't need me, but she wanted me to come east and share in the wonder of dear Cait. I was desperate to get there and experience the joy firsthand.

I created a trip to New York via Boston. Phil gladly spent several days with Jena while I flew on to New York City alone. Oliver was called out of town on business, so I was actually needed for support. I slept on the couch in their tiny apartment and spent endless minutes just smiling into the face of the sweet babe. Beth and I practiced taking her on outings to Central Park and learned how to manage the stroller/infant seat/cab routine to venture to Soho for lunch. Adventure and appreciation filled my heart.

Jena and Phil then flew in to meet Cait too. Phil was full of stories about his Boston time with the big grandchildren and Jena's loading his new iPod with 540 songs. He chattered away as Jena scooped up Cait for her brief two-hour stay. I wanted to get Phil to bed on schedule, so I excused us after supper, saying, "We need to watch the presidential debate." We walked hand in hand to a nearby hotel, pulling his roller suitcase.

We stayed one more day. Rested, Grandpa was ready to push the stroller across the Brooklyn Bridge for pizza. Daddy Oliver was home. The tender feeling of this new family engulfed us. Phil was thrilled to have his turn; the rest of us were equally glad for his chance to fill up on family love.

A progressive disease, Alzheimer's was on the march, causing Phil to stumble more frequently socially. His inappropriate remarks with strangers didn't really matter, but his unpleasant attitude with good friends did—at least to me. He seemed more comfortable with people he didn't know, chatting freely without struggling to make sense.

Our annual visit to the American Craft Show with the Kiernats in April did not suit him. Instead of coming in the house to get ready to go when I asked, he lit the brush in our burning pit. There was no time to tend a fire. My helping put it out was not what he wanted. When we arrived at the meeting place, he protested, "Look at all the purses. This is a women's show!" Bruce smiled and said, "Come on, Phil, let's go have a cup of coffee." In prior years Phil had enjoyed the juried art and craft show. Phil was snarly and unpersuaded by Bruce to let us women have a moment of fun. His impatience forced us to leave in less than a half hour.

The Roy women were planning a brief New York City rendezvous in May to include Jena, Heidi, Heidi's little girls, pregnant Beth, baby Cait, and me. I didn't feel comfortable leaving Phil alone while I joined the gang in New York. I certainly didn't want him to light a fire. As talk of the possible trip ensued, Phil encouraged me to go. Mostly, I needed to give myself permission to do it and arrange a support system for Phil's enjoyment.

"I have to care for the dogs," he reminded me. I spoke plainly, "Taking your medication is very important and easily forgotten." He accepted my point as a fact, not a chastisement. In the end, Phil agreed to have Bruce partner with him. They planned to do some fishing and walk their dogs together.

Once on my way, I felt a kind of weightlessness, flying into the bosom of the Roy women. We called Phil daily, and Beth delighted him with the news of her second pregnancy. Cheerful connections persisted until my return flight was delayed. When I called to explain the change, Phil was agitated—perhaps by the length of my being away, by the change in my schedule, by two days of rain at home, by the long, faithful care of Bruce, by irregular consumption of his medication. In any case he was worried about a yard project and contacting a carpenter. I spent ten minutes walking him through finding the phone numbers he wanted in our directory. When I arrived several hours late, Phil turned to Bruce and directed him, "Go home!"

With Phil's approval, I had bought advance tickets for us and the Kiernats to attend a tribute to Frank Sinatra the night after I got back from New York. In my mind the event would be a festive thank-you to our friends. Phil was rude at dinner. "Bruce, you are not funny!" he complained. Further Phil asserted that Bruce talked too much. The concert's familiar songs did not perk him up; he fell asleep. His effort to get along without me had taken a toll. Privately, Sandy and Bruce assured me that they did not take Phil's grumpiness personally.

Phil and I needed quiet time by ourselves. That summer of 2005 I concentrated on finding a balance between interesting activity and passive relaxation for us. Phil was not much of a sitter. One Saturday after attending Wayne Caron's support group at the university, Phil suggested going to Gerten's Nursery to look around. We came home with four junipers that had appealed to him. My thoughts raced in considering where to plant and how to make the planting experience pleasant. I knew where I didn't want them: scattered willy-nilly wherever Phil's fancy struck, such as in the middle of the yard. We walked around and placed reflective markers at suitable planting sites. I assembled buckets, shovels, and rakes, while Phil wheelbarrowed the heavy pots into position. With the hose running and mulch at hand, we were ready.

The first dig included removing some prairie grasses that I could replant later. I put the clumps in one of the wheelbarrows. We watered the hole, plopped the juniper in, backfilled around it, encircled it with mulch, and watered it some more.

The pattern for successful planting did not last. Phil spread the mulch before the next hole was dug. When he did dig the hole, he dumped the excavated dirt into the wheelbarrow containing the prairie grass collection. Oblivious to redirection, he grabbed the hose and further filled the wheelbarrow with water, smothering the prairie grass in mud. The goofy sequence felt as if we were in a Three Stooges comedy act. I'd never been a fan of slapstick, and I hated being cast in one. This show didn't have an intermission; it was unrelenting!

Once the junipers were finally in the ground, Phil stomped into the house wearing his mud-caked tennis shoes. Our desperation in trying to hang onto life as we had known it was making him aggressive and crabby and me frustrated and sad. I was left to pick up strewn gardening equipment and consider his mess-in-the-making. I didn't chase after Phil to insist that he remove his shoes. Instead, I slumped on the grass, wishing he'd felt some pleasure in our work together. Crafting any project that we could do together was growing impossible. My desire to respect Phil's feelings while having to think for both of us was taking a personal toll. I could barely keep up in the confusion.

He often lamented, "I have nothing to do." Sometimes I offered no immediate solution. Some of my suggestions were unappealing to him. He did willingly ride along on errands, but complained if the drive was too long. "You're trapping me into a stiff position," he would say. Occasionally he was ready for dinner by four—not because he was hungry but because there was nothing more to do. We faithfully watched the local 5 p.m. news followed by the Lehrer *NewsHour* at six. Then the evening loomed. Playing games did not work well. Watching more TV often bored me. Conversation was difficult.

One night I excused myself to take some Tylenol for a headache. Phil put the dogs in the kennel and followed me to the bedroom. "Phil, I have to admit that I'm exhausted," I told him. In tender language and the simplest terms I could find, I also tried to get across that his despair was difficult for me as well, that my responses to him were imperfect but well intended, that deconstructing my own daily tasks to communicate what I was doing all the time was hard, that making social plans was complicated by not knowing what might suit when the time came, and that I cared deeply about him.

Phil caught my emotional tone, kissed me, and offered words of appreciation. Knowingly he said, "Would you like to read for a while?" Ordinarily my reading annoyed him because he felt it shut him out. He was conceding me some personal pleasure.

I knew, even though I didn't like to admit it to myself, that Phil was slipping. At our next appointment with Dr. Holm, he asked us how things were different. I described Phil's tirade with a Schwan's delivery-man who'd stopped in our driveway to inquire if we might like service. Phil banished him. On a walk later, Phil spotted the Schwan's truck on another street. He gestured at the driver and yelled, "Get out of here!"

In another instance, Phil had become angry when our phone rang and angrier yet when I took it to my desk to check something on the calendar. He had misinterpreted my taking the phone as "running away." Phil weighed in indifferently, unable to marshal any further description or personal explanation.

Dr. Holm's three areas of concern for us were: environment, medication, and mood. His emphasis on the complexity of our home environment really concerned me. "Phil has to work very hard to live in it," he told us. I knew I was working very hard to build routine and yet preserve some enrichment. Safety was important. The fire pit needed to go, but what else? I couldn't make the garage disappear. We'd given away the power tools and sold the tiller and lawn mower to the landscape service.

Remaining hoses and watering cans seemed safe. Most importantly, I'd secretly transferred all Phil's hunting guns to Heidi's gun safe. I began to worry that Dr. Holm was referring to ordinary stuff. Did we have too many utensils in the kitchen, too many beauty products in the bathroom, too many clickers for the TVs, too many clothes in Phil's closet?

Phil was slated to play golf the next morning. When we got ready for bed that night, he wanted to keep his golf shirt on so he'd be ready. I convinced him to let me wash it and his chinos even though he no longer liked to change his clothes. After the doctor's visit, I was more conscious that changing his clothes was hard work for Phil. When he stripped, he had on two pairs of boxers. He'd probably forgotten which pair he'd meant to put in the laundry the day before and which pair was fresh.

I received other, nonprofessional feedback too. My brother came through town. "Barbara, you look like hell!" he said frankly but lovingly. Phil's sister Allie came up from Dallas to see her brother. She was not as candid about my appearance, but she reasserted the message. "You need to take care of yourself," she said. She was deeply sad to see Phil as a shell of his former self, but she didn't want us both to go down. "Get some respite help!" she urged.

Beth was due with her second baby on November 10. I knew I wasn't going to be able to leave Phil for the birth. What I hadn't anticipated was that Imogen would arrive prematurely, that her daddy would be in Boston on business, and that a Northeaster would be threatening to close the airport. One-year-old Cait ended up in the care of a slightly known condo neighbor, and Beth went to the hospital on her own.

Phil and I had been at a funeral with my cell phone turned off. I checked for messages before driving home. My motherly heart sank, hearing my daughter's voice. She was in labor, alone, and 1,500 miles away. There was nothing I could do to help. I looked at Phil in despair, hating the disease that prevented my rushing east.

Beth was able to call us again just as we arrived home. She confirmed that Oliver was on the way to take care of Cait. "I can manage having this baby on my own," she declared. I was so glad to hear her voice that I didn't argue with her bravado. On the face of it she could and would manage. She promised Oliver would call us when he landed. She was on medication to slow contractions until four p.m., when she could have her final penicillin shot to support the baby's health. Click.

I called Heidi. She quickly picked up on everyone's emotional turmoil. More family support was needed in New York. If I couldn't go, then she would. In no time she made arrangements for her own family and booked herself on the six p.m. flight to LaGuardia.

When Oliver called from a New York taxi, I told him, "Heidi will be there at ten p.m.!" At Beth's insistence he went straight to the condo to rescue Cait and tuck her in for the night. The kind neighbor returned to await Heidi's arrival, and Oliver finally hurried to the hospital. Imogen waited for her daddy before being born, and the three of them spent the night together. Oliver immediately began a two-week paternity leave. Heidi stayed until Beth came home from the hospital, reassuring everyone that Imogen's prescribed ten-day stay there was merely a precaution to oversee her lung development.

I felt so disconnected and far away. My dear friend Lynn offered to teach me to knit so I could make Imogen a blanket. The pattern required me to pay attention. Working on my own, I naturally made a mistake and then didn't know how to repair it. I sighed and made an executive decision to accept mistakes as part of the piece. The blanket was still hanging together. I worked on it in the evenings while Phil watched TV. I enjoyed the blanket's growing weight in my lap and the tactile metaphor of living with imperfection. The gaps and bumps in it represented my personal, variable tension and lots of love.

Allie called with congratulations. She insisted that she was taking off a few days from work so that she could return to Minnesota. She wanted me to go to New York to help Beth after Imogen came home from the hospital.

Phil was not supportive this time. Medication changes were helping his mood somewhat, but he was still irritable. To him, I never seemed to think of anything fun to do, I didn't do a good job of explaining what I meant, and I made him work too hard. And yet he didn't want to get rid of me. In fact, he didn't want me out of his sight! But I needed a time-out.

Before taking my leave, I slowed our pace another notch, trying

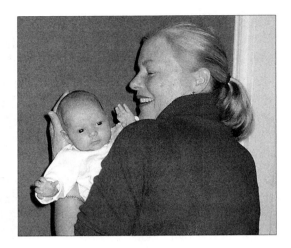

*Me holding Imogen*

to keep the peace. Abby and Ken invited us for supper, a balm that diluted Phil's and my intense togetherness. Phil was able to talk about Allie's upcoming visit and my trip to New York to help Beth. We both enthused about our future trip to Boston over Thanksgiving. Just having these plans lifted my spirits considerably.

Once I was away, my concern for the Minnesota front faded. Morning and nightly check-ins brought news but affirmed my suspended responsibility. Heidi and Allie were taking loving charge, using their imaginations to enliven and ease Phil's existence. Each day Beth and I went on long, energetic walks with the double stroller. We had quiet time in the evening to chat. We did not dwell on the circumstance of Phil's and my life, but we did address it openly and honestly. Tears of understanding and bewilderment slipped down Beth's cheek. Deep mother-daughter closeness lent mutual support to both of our new roles.

When I returned to Phil, he was anxious for our Thanksgiving trip to Boston. I packed for both of us. Jena picked us up at Logan Airport. As we'd done the previous Christmas, he and I grocery-shopped from Jena's list. Seated at the big work island in her kitchen, Phil gladly watched food preparation. He helped carry boxes to the car for the drive to Vermont. With snow in the forecast, we stopped to buy long underwear and again at a farm to collect a twenty-five-pound, free-range turkey. Phil was happily on point and on task.

On Thanksgiving morning snow was accumulating—the marvel of first snow yet another element to be thankful for. A fire blazed in the farmhouse fireplace. With the bird in the oven, we all took a walk on unplowed country roads toward Woodstock. My camera captured frame after frame of exquisite scene and family frolic. Bella, the family dog, stuck her snout in every drift. Safe and loved, Phil and I were in charge of nothing and the beneficiaries of so much, a true Thanksgiving blessing and awareness.

# CHAPTER 7

# Preserving Phil's Story

With Alzheimer's escalating, we continued to ride a roller coaster of highs and lows. Ordinary living was rarely ordinary any more. The 2005 Thanksgiving in Vermont was a definite high. During that year I had begun to face the truth that Phil's life story was losing its base. All that he'd been and done was fading for him.

On July 9, 2005, Phil turned sixty-five, the age when people take stock of their accomplishments and, if lucky, begin new lives based on their experience and dreams. Phil had retired early. Our dreams were in tatters. Taking stock was hard for him. He was losing a wonderful story of what had been important to him, what he'd learned, and how his life changed. I wanted to help him hold onto his memories as long as he could. I despaired of Alzheimer's undefining Phil somehow. I cherished his former vitality and unique experience.

I decided to commemorate his birthday in a special way. Years before we'd attended a St. Croix Valley pottery show, where we'd both admired the work of Amy Sabrina. Her ceramic pieces were beautiful to look at, and many were also ceremonial. She accepted commissions for personalized bowls that she called BioGraphic Pottery. They were painted with twenty-four window-like panels, each representing a key element in the honored person's life. I imagined Phil might relate to his life depicted on such a bowl and decided to contact her. I hoped her colorful images could cue Phil's memory of himself.

I learned that not only was she an artist but she also saw herself as a spiritual healer. She insisted on knowing her subject to inspire her creation. To preserve the surprise for Phil, I scheduled Amy's face-to-face interview with me during one of his outings with Bruce Kiernat. She drove from Dalbo, Minnesota, to our home in St. Mary's Point to get a sense of our setting and lifestyle. Together we went over my preliminary list of possible subjects, such as his alma maters, army service, surgery, love of hockey and orchids, yard projects, dogs, hunting and fishing, travel and boating on the St. Croix River, and golf. For travel I came up with the image of a Mounds candy bar, which Phil always bought in the airport before we boarded a plane. Buckled in and ready for adventure, he would produce the treat to share. I enjoyed telling Amy about Phil's passions and unique qualities. Our thoughtful time together produced a carefully chosen set of twenty-four subjects for the panels around Phil's bowl.

Amy had brought her camera to record aspects of our life at home. When I described Phil's handyman status and perpetual productivity, she asked me to photograph his hands and send her the picture. Phil was used to my picture taking, so several days later, when I asked him to stick out his paws during a stump removal project, he just submitted to the request. The earth embedded in his nails became a wonderful reminder of his pleasure in being a dirtball.

Many months after the interview, Amy called to say Phil's bowl was ready. I agreed to meet at a Dairy Queen halfway between Dalbo and our home. Phil was willing to go for a drive. "I need to pick up a box of annual reports for the Wilder Foundation," I explained. I'd grown accustomed to therapeutic lying.

As long as I kept my voice cheerful and my story uncomplicated, Phil was accepting. He was not suspicious of this strange meeting place. I set Amy's unopened box carefully into the trunk, ordered Phil and me cones dipped in chocolate, and turned the car back onto the highway.

I could hardly wait to sneak a peek at Amy's creation after Phil went to sleep that night. It shone as an art object, but more importantly it paid tribute to my man. I turned it slowly and ran my fingers over the images. I could see Phil touching the quail window and streaming whatever that image evoked for him. I wanted others to know what was important to Phil and what he could still talk about. Deep inside I knew that the bowl would stay with me longer than Phil could. It would be my memory bowl too.

The finished piece included Amy's close-up of the starter's handle on Phil's orange and white Stihl chainsaw. She framed our Brittany spaniel Lily's freckled nose and adoring eye. Our John Deere Gator 4x2 showed the baby seat that Phil had rigged up on the passenger side for Sunny. Phil's simple aqua surgery shirt was in the panel next to the complex composition of our boat going backwards under the Prescott Lift Bridge. A delicate, white orchid contrasted with buckthorn leaves in a red circle with a slash through it. The Jupiter Lighthouse in Florida recalled our pleasant nights of eating yellowtail snapper at the Jetty across the waterway from the famous landmark. An ordinarily tiny dry fly for trout fishing was depicted as big as the army major insignia. Her whole presentation turned out perfectly.

The morning of Phil's birthday I presented my special gift, unsure what he'd make of it. I showed him the small black and white plate we'd purchased from Amy at the pottery show. "She's the one who made those colorful bowls with all the pictures. Look at this," I encouraged.

Phil began to see that the images on the bowl were about him. I turned the bowl over and showed him the inscription: "To PHIL on your 65th birthday, July 9, 2005. Love always, Barbara." He was

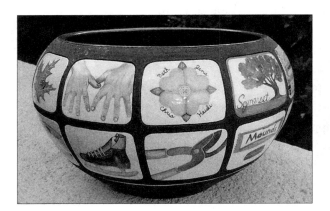

*Phil's bowl*

touched, and I was thrilled. A lot of thought, work, and waiting had gone into this moment, but it paid off.

That night several couples came to our home for dinner to celebrate Phil's birthday. He proudly showed them his bowl. He could initiate conversation, pointing to each picture to tell his own stories. Our friends easily followed his lead. I loved seeing him in command of his former experience. The memory cues were working.

The sad truth was that Phil's ability to converse was slipping rapidly. He still had language, but the word combinations were strange. His zany Robin Williams sense of humor and antics covered some of his nonsense, but getting a serious idea across was a challenge for him.

We went to see Wayne Caron for private lessons in hopes of being able to talk to one another more easily. I had always enjoyed laughing at and with Phil, but silliness could not be our only satisfying mode of communication. Unfortunately, Phil was clearest when he was angry. He knew what he didn't like, and that expression came easily. I wanted to hear more than complaints and protests. Wayne suggested working together on a story of Phil's life.

With the golf season winding down, the days growing darker, and outdoor projects more difficult to identify, a writing project was a fresh idea. I tried to get Phil to talk about himself, a concrete subject about which he knew a lot. I hoped to sketch a traditional account of his life story that the whole family could keep.

Phil knew that I'd worked previously with my mom in Florida to document some of her personal history. Back in 2003, while Phil had played golf on men's day, I had interviewed Mother. She was a great storyteller. I barely needed a question to set her in motion. I scribbled notes to take back to our condo, entered the segment into my computer, faxed the piece to her for corrections, and reappeared the next Tuesday for more of the same. In the end, we added some historical photos, and I took the works to Kinko's to be transformed into a booklet. The piece wasn't long, and Phil had read it.

He seemed glad for his own turn. I spent numerous, after-breakfast sessions listening to snippets about his growing up in St. Paul. He willingly talked about his childhood, school days, and family of origin.

Sometimes his eyes would brim with tears, but he was not able to articulate his feelings. Gently drawing him out, I heard few new details, but from the ones he repeated over and over again I gleaned what was important to him. His mother had been extremely proud of him, taking him to her Episcopal church and enlisting him as a caddy for her golf games. He recalled her saying, "Here's my boy!" He reported working hard at his studies and team sports. He liked his college fraternity but felt uncomfortable with some of the wealthy guys who played Monopoly with real money. He loved the live music on party weekends.

He talked a bit about his career in medicine. I reminded him that he'd been president of the Ramsey County Medical Society and an alternate delegate to the AMA. What mattered more to him were the patients, their problems, their recoveries, and in some cases their demise. His delight in helping people was clear. He remembered drawing pictures of the procedures he recommended and offering a light joke when the surgery was over. After retirement, all of us in the family had continued to bump into former patients who expressed their appreciation for his care. One gentleman phoned our home, not knowing of Phil's illness. He was going to see the new World War II Memorial in Washington, DC, and wanted Phil to know he'd taken his advice after surgery fifteen years earlier: "Go home and lead your life." He was so excited to have made it to this historic moment as a veteran.

We talked about being grandparents and what our kids were up to. Phil told me somewhat impatiently, "You know all this stuff." What I wanted was his perspective, but I was unsuccessful in teasing out his unique experience in our family. That we all belonged to each other was the main thing to him. He kept repeating the word "heritage."

Along the way random remarks in our many conversations spotlighted the limited but important times we invested in play and recreation. The other theme that emerged was Phil's love of the land wherever he lived. From being a teenage greens keeper at Town and Country Club to his retirement in our wildflower meadow, Phil was a steward of the land. I well knew his urge to get outside and get to work.

At night when Phil would fall asleep watching TV in bed, I would slip into my adjacent office and turn my notes into pieces of his story.

Eventually, I presented the narrative, reading it aloud for his approval. He offered no corrections or objections.

Listening, however, Phil filled up anew. In the preface I explained the impetus for his storytelling: his value on heritage, Wayne Caron's encouragement, and my pleasure in writing. I told prospective readers: "Phil's life so far is offered here in appreciation for all that he's known and participated in. He has a grateful heart!"

We combed through old photo albums and selected pertinent pictures that suited Phil's story. Phil was anxious to go to Kinko's to print his book. He stood beside me for two hours while I printed the material and put together ten books. Under the clear plastic cover I used a large picture of Phil with his dogs, Lily and Sunny. His name in large capitals, PHILEMON CHEVERTON ROY, JUNIOR, MD, was the simple title.

We took the copies to the post office to mail to out-of-town family members and ran into Heidi. Phil personally presented a book to her. They leafed through it together, while I weighed the mailing envelopes. The photographs in each section helped Phil tell her some of the contents. "Here's my family's house in St. Paul," he showed her. Heidi could see that he was proud of the product.

I wasn't sure how it would be received across the family. Our objective was certainly not to present some kind of elongated obituary or powder keg of emotional grief. I relegated Alzheimer's to the preface; it had no place in the body of the story. I hoped our children might find interesting the things their dad was doing at their ages. Some of the historical pictures would be new to them.

In the end, the piece disappeared into the confusion of the Christmas holidays. The children said, "Thank you," and that was it. The whole exercise had been for Phil and me, a way to savor the remnants of our verbal communication and true understanding.

I longed for the intimacy of being known by my beloved and discovering every day more of who he was. That possibility was evaporating day by day. I had to be satisfied with my own memories. Dear Phil was barely holding onto his.

# CHAPTER 8

# Falling Apart

The jig was up. By 2006 I had become a visible caregiver. Neither Phil nor I was happy with the situation. Phil's zest was disappearing, and my spirits were low. He complained about the phone ringing, the disposal grinding, the mixer whirring as I made dinner. He said the noises disturbed his reading. The magazine was in pieces, discarded pages ripped out as he reviewed it—his reading was no longer really reading. I knew he liked to keep me in his sight, and I also knew my nerves were fraying.

One afternoon, my good friend Abby called to check up on me. As I picked up the phone, Phil griped, "Who's calling now?" I read the caller ID and said, "It's Ab." He fumed while I chatted briefly. Hanging up, I lost my temper and shouted at him, "I will not let you shut me down. I will speak on the phone when someone calls!"

We needed to break out of our funk. We were no longer candidates for a Lindblad Expedition with strangers. Instead I envisioned visiting Phil's sister in Dallas for a simple family affair. My idea was to surprise Allie for her sixtieth birthday in February. We called sister Barbie in Detroit and stepmom Sally in California, asking them to join the fun. Allie's husband and children coordinated the event at the local level. Phil perked up.

Allie's surprise in seeing us all in her daughter's living room and the subsequent family dinner in a private room at a fine restaurant were wonderful. Phil exuded love for his clan. I did not cancel the single scotch he ordered himself. I had his credit card ready so he could pay for the party as he wished to do. We all went to bed tired and happy.

Day 2 began with the Roy siblings drinking coffee at the kitchen table. We went back to niece Sarah's for brunch at ten. That party broke up at the children's naptime. The sixty-and-over crowd returned to Allie's to go for a walk and watch the Olympics on TV. Phil sat with his sister Barbie on the couch and fell asleep. I didn't pay much attention to him. At five we were to go out for Mexican fare. No one was drinking. The atmosphere was very relaxed.

The worm turned, however, around four thirty, when I suggested to Phil that we get ready to leave again. He was unsteady on his feet. I thought perhaps he was stiff from sitting so long. He was angry when I mentioned tucking in his shirttail. He didn't know where our room was in the house. On hearing he was in the wrong bedroom, he grabbed a bottle of perfume and threw it across the room. I'd never seen him act like this.

Suddenly it dawned on me that he might have been drinking. There was an open bar in the den. I asked him. Of course, he denied drinking. He said something nasty to Allie. She told him to apologize. He pinned her against the wall. His happy world was collapsing in on him. The agitation and combativeness were typical of Alzheimer's, but this time they were extreme.

I told the family that Phil and I would stay behind. Fortunately Allie's husband, Rich, and Chad, Sarah's husband, insisted on staying home as well. Rich confirmed that the scotch bottle on the bar was low. Phil's behavior escalated. He threw a dried flower arrangement on the floor, pushed Rich, and swung at Chad. He lurched into the kitchen and smashed two dishes. The men tried to get him outside for "fresh air." I called 911. I told the operator that my husband was out of control and suffering from Alzheimer's, and had likely drunk an undetermined amount of scotch.

First the police came; then the paramedics arrived. They restrained Phil. As he sat on the lawn, his wrists secured by plastic ties behind his back, he vehemently cursed them. Looking directly at me, he roared, "I'm done with you forever." I rode up front in the emergency vehicle; I could hear him thrashing and raging against the attendants. At the emergency room of the Baylor Regional Medical Center, he was restrained to the bed. I approved a shot of Ativan to try to bring him down. He wanted to see everyone's credentials. In a vain attempt to assert his authority, he told the staff that he was a doctor and had served in Vietnam.

He kicked one of the nurses, so off came his tennis shoes. A police officer and a nurse, who was a former college football player, stayed in the room. When the medicine began to work, the two men and I tried to talk Phil down. Unfortunately, the police officer took off the restraints prematurely. Phil ripped out his IV, spurting blood all over the room. The restraints had to be reapplied, which started the ordeal all over again. The nurse straddled Phil's legs. Two other nurses came to help. Phil grabbed one of their stethoscopes and swung it threateningly. He clutched the other's head in a hammerlock. I approved a shot of Haldol. We waited for its effect. Meanwhile, the test came back showing that his blood alcohol level was elevated.

I stayed out of the room until Phil told the nurses he wanted to see me. I caressed his head and told him that the scotch had poisoned him, that he couldn't be released until it cleared his system, and that I would sleep in the room with him. He relaxed with the medication and dozed. He never knew that Rich and Sally stopped in to see him. Shortly after midnight we were given a room on a medical unit, where he remained restrained to the bed rails. I wrapped up in a blanket and slept fitfully on a pullout couch. I was too tired to think how we would get back to Minnesota.

At home, I felt guilty for not being able to foresee that I was attempting too much. In trying to entertain Phil and honor his love of family, I'd exhausted him. Checking in with our professionals, I found little comfort in psychologist Wayne Caron's easy explanation. "You've experienced a *catastrophic incident*, Barbara. These things happen in families caring for a member with dementing illness." He acted as if our incident was ordinary, to be expected, and no big deal. Certainly accepting absurdity and laughing had been important before. Wayne's emphasis on the whole person and a family-oriented approach to dementia had served us well in the past. In the Dallas mess I saw nothing to laugh about.

Unhappy with Wayne's attempt to soothe me, I turned to Dr. Holm, whose expertise was disease, not family systems. He reminded me that people with Alzheimer's were hypersensitive to stimulation. The party weekend in Texas might have contributed as much as the alcohol to Phil's upset. He also said that Phil's violent behavior might be a precursor of things to come. His point of view was not soothing, but it gave me a course of action: stay home, and keep life simple.

Phil did not remember his trip to a hospital in Dallas, a blessing for him. Once home, I curtailed social outings. We even stopped going for walks in the following weeks. An occasional errand allowed us to replenish our cupboard and have the birthday photos developed. Phil pushed the grocery cart with no complaints. He wanted to get the photos back. Riding in the car, he dozed. Watching Olympic hockey games in the afternoon, he nodded off. Watching more TV after dinner, he fell asleep. He allowed me to put the dogs in their garage kennel at night, a job he usually did. He did not want to be bothered taking off his corduroys before getting into bed. He was wiped.

My response was a doozie of a cold. My eyes became slits. Wearing Phil's sweatpants and a huge wool turtleneck over my pajamas, I looked sicker than Phil in the bathroom mirror. With rest, Phil gradually became more cheerful, and I recovered from debilitating congestion. What was our new normal to be? For sure, it included no drinking and no travel.

Interestingly, Phil did not object to the loss of a drink. Heidi had removed all liquor from our house before we returned from Texas. Its absence erased its existence somehow. Phil didn't see the bottles, he didn't see anyone drinking, and having a beer didn't occur to him. Months later, when we met friends for dinner in town, I asked them in advance not to order a cocktail or wine. On another occasion, his hunting buddies had a small party and omitted liquor so we could come. I did not sign us up for the golf club opening dinner that included celebratory drinks. I reasoned that if Phil saw others drinking, he would want to join in, rather like a kid wanting the candy he saw others enjoying.

Living in a teetotalling household was a relief to me. As our in-house barkeep, Phil had long before lost his skill to measure one ounce, and he confused the tonic and soda. I had poured many of his concoctions down the drain. Before the Dallas trip, I hadn't removed the bar contents, however, because he would have squawked in fierce opposition, demanding, "What are you doing?" Instead I had created a routine of his having one beer before supper. I had never acquired the taste, preferring wine myself. My one glass of wine did not empty a bottle, and I didn't want Phil to finish it, so I left our wine in the cupboard. Too much alcohol had worried me. Finding a kind and decisive way to say no to Phil was a tiresome job. Removing the alcohol altogether solved a lot of problems.

Our days of doing little were nonetheless tiring. I tried to get a good night's sleep. One night I dreamed about driving in the country and stopping at an unfamiliar property. It was a lovely day. I parked the car at a detached garage and walked around the building toward the house. Behind the garage I came upon a mountainous pile of gravel. In the dream I thought, "I didn't order that. Did Phil? I don't want that ugly stuff." I stormed, "What will I do with it?" I looked around to assure myself that nothing further spoiled the natural setting. Then I saw exposed earth and ripped roots making a crude path from the house into the woods. I couldn't see where it went in the thicket. In stunned silence I looked from the pile to the path and sighed, "If that gravel is supposed to be the road bed for that new path, there is no way I can move it into place by myself." Waking up, I knew the dream was a warning of sorts: I needed to stay alert not just emotionally but practically to change.

After the Dallas catastrophe, our children were also on high alert. We planned a family meeting with Wayne Caron to assess where we were in the Alzheimer's journey. The children insisted that the meeting be without Phil so everyone could speak plainly. I mailed them a copy of a chapter on behavior from Wayne's book, *Alzheimer's Disease: The Family Journey*. Beth made a stab at some goals and objectives for the meeting. Heidi did homework on community resources. I hoped just being all together in conversation would have value in and of itself. How to engage Phil in some way that allowed all of us to escape to the university was an epiphany yet to come.

I wrote down my questions for the meeting:

1. How are we doing? How is Phil doing? How am I doing?
2. What are the children's concerns?
3. What kind of help do we need?
4. How do we avoid more catastrophic incidents?
5. Under what circumstances would Phil be better cared for not at home?
6. How can we preserve the fun in family relations?
7. How can I get away to see the out-of-town family members (including my ninety-four-year-old mother, now living in Texas with my brother)?
8. How long will Phil's decline go on? What might be expected next?
9. What kind of balance can be struck in honoring Phil and nourishing my being?
10. What's the genetic reality of Phil's disease?

Then I wrote down what I thought I knew in response to the questions at that point in March 2006.

1. Phil's and my relationship is strong. He can be cheerful. I am tired.
2. The children want us to be safe and me to have some time off from caregiving.
3. We need and use informal help from friends. We are trying a new arrangement with a woman coming to the house a half day a week to partner with Phil and allow me to work in my office.
4. I need to keep life as simple and routine as I can.
5. If Phil becomes violent or physically incapacitated, or if he doesn't know us, then professionals might better care for him.
6. Family coming to Minnesota is a boon to my spirits.
7. Jena is willing to set aside a week to come home and be the in-house caregiver so I can get away. We have a contingency plan to admit Phil to Bethesda Hospital for in-patient assessment if he becomes too agitated.

8.  Phil's physical health is good.
9.  I've lost my sense of proportion.
10. Mayo Clinic told me not to worry about genetics. We still do!

I knew that one meeting would not completely or finally answer all of our questions, but I was anxious to hear what Wayne would have to say to us.

Phil and I spent the next month in slow motion. There were two big dumps of snow. Our short-legged dogs needed snorkels to go outside to pee. Phil and I enjoyed the pristine scene mostly from the window. I had the driveway plowed by a truck. We listened to books on CD. I learned about George Washington, Teddy Roosevelt, the Panama Canal, and Abraham Lincoln's *Team of Rivals*. Phil sat willingly for story hour. Seeing me relax seemed to help him do the same. One night I had an affirming dream: I was on a dock, very content. In the water I noticed an alligator eye blinking in the sun. Then I saw more alligators and was glad I had not jumped in for a swim. Surrendering to the snowstorms and Phil's limitations had surprised me with a feeling of contentment despite lurking trouble.

Chris had recently completed his master's degree at the University of Montana. The children planned a celebration of his achievement in part as a cover for their coming to town for our upcoming meeting with Wayne. Our friend Tom Kingston, president of the Wilder Foundation, developed a great diversion so the children and I could go to the meeting. He invited Phil to ride along to Wilder Forest and inspect the buildings, designed by the same architect who had done our house. Phil was delighted to be of help. We excused him for his important assignment, saying we'd celebrate Chris at dinner. Undaunted by a rainstorm, Phil and Tom left in high spirits. The children and I were able to escape and return before the men did.

We began our meeting by going around the circle to say why we were there. Heidi started. "I love Dad, though growing up I didn't like him being such a clown." She admitted that it was hard for her to set a plan, get a babysitter, and have me cancel it. She had been promoting day care for her dad, and I had struggled to find the right time for the experiment. I was next and immediately dissolved into tears. I managed to say, "I miss our easy conversations and ordinary fun." Jena said it was hard to be so far away geographically. She hoped we could listen to each other and be authentic. Beth offered, "I love Mom and feel sorry for Dad." She wanted an action plan to address the circumstance. Chris paused. "I'm the least articulate," he began, but then expressed his desire to be present to the situation. He felt he'd been out of the loop until the flurry of urgent emails in recent months. "I'm somewhat shocked that we are now talking about plans for Dad's care."

Wayne poked at me. "Barbara, you are very controlling." That felt lousy. In my mind, I had been trying darn hard to make Phil's life as bright as possible. The girls chipped in their truth: "It's so hard to go back to the old days, when Mom always seemed to put Dad first." One of them said, "He was so self-centered!" Chris, the youngest by five years, looked confused. Beth was direct. "Mom, you have no life. You've given up everything and everyone except Dad." Wayne liked the anger, telling me, "You do not have a very good poker face, Barbara." I didn't. Underneath I must have wanted the children to see me as I felt, worn out and insufficient. I promised to try day care the following week and to aim at ramping up to two days a week.

Wayne counseled that memory care assisted living was best considered outside of crisis and didn't end the family's caregiving. He told us, "Doing the homework to assess the resources and scheduling placement are weighty tasks that can best be done with a lot of mutual support." He encouraged us to reframe our thinking from looking for signs of deterioration that necessitated placing Phil to thinking what was actually best for Phil. In the new frame, Wayne pointed out three key factors: (1) It's okay for Phil to be unhappy sometimes, and he will be more so as time goes along. (2) Day care and memory care units are not necessarily negative confinements; they can also provide sociability and less stressful environments. (3) While Phil can connect with others, he is more likely to be socially successful in another setting.

The outcome of the meeting was not immediately satisfying because all of our choices seemed too hard—too hard on Phil psychologically, too hard for me to enact, and perhaps too long overdue.

Phil was already growing weary of the wonderful woman I'd hired to do things with him a half day a week. I tried to set them up for success by telling Phil how much he was helping me and giving them defined tasks. They walked the dogs in a nearby park. They went to the grocery store. I thanked Phil profusely for doing these chores so I could tend our business at my desk. Eventually, however, he rebelled at having Jean come into his house or drive his car. His frustration and unease were palpable.

Heidi took the lead to introduce Phil to Circle of Friends, an adult day program in nearby Stillwater. Anticipating their trial anguished me. Phil was still strong; there was no making him do anything he was unwilling to do. Heidi casually showed him the site. He didn't really understand that it was a care program for him. The director was cordial. Unfortunately, the required assessment drew Phil's alarm when he couldn't answer the questions. Heidi covered: "Don't worry, Dad. I had to fill out that sort of paperwork before I could volunteer at Afton Lakeland School. Let me help you." She signed him up to return the next week.

On the appointed day, Heidi came to get Phil, took him into the program, and left him there. She wanted me to get some exercise and let go of Phil. I was to pick him up at three thirty, after I played golf. I took our dog Mariah with me for the pick up. She pranced into the facility, earning Phil's smile and everyone's attention. Phil was so pleased to see us that he did not immediately launch into his despairing tale of being abandoned. On the way home, Chris called to tell us that he'd successfully defended his thesis. That happy news trumped any simmering angst.

Over dinner Phil and I discussed his day. "I didn't know Heidi was going to leave me. Where were you?" he asked, annoyed. He was adamant that he would never go there again. I changed the subject, hoping he would forget his negative stance. I was still high from my experience of getting him off successfully (showered, fed, and eager to partner with Heidi), disciplining myself not to pick him up before three thirty, avoiding upset at pickup, and having six hours to myself. I clung to Wayne's admonition: "It's okay if Phil is unhappy sometimes."

The night before Phil was to return, I brought up Circle of Friends. He smelled my anxiety. "I told you I am *not* ever going to THAT PLACE again." I tried to be firm with him: "Your having a social time allows me to play golf." He didn't see it that way: "People just stare into space. There's nothing to do!" The phone rang. It was Heidi, who asked "Are you set for tomorrow?" I was stuck.

I botched the communication. Maybe I should have waited until the morning and taken my chance on compliance. Instead, I had fired Phil's defiance. The only good news was that he did not know that he was supposed to go the next day. I didn't want him to think I might cave in to him. If he went, it would be his second day that week. I skipped it.

Several days later we went to Heidi's for a family supper. She found a moment to speak with her dad and apologized for any misunderstanding regarding her part in taking him to Circle of Friends. Phil accepted her apology without rancor, making clear that the social group was not a good fit for him. Heidi listened. I was surprised that she let it go so easily. I had not yet let him off the hook for the following Tuesday, my golf day. His reservation was still in place at day care.

Heidi called the next morning. She was back on course: "We'll never know if the program works if we don't persevere." She wanted to try again. I agreed. Phil had no idea of her change of heart or what day he was expected to return. He was in a particularly tender mood, offering me shoulder rubs and enjoying a shared project of assembling Adirondack chairs. As far as he was concerned, life was good.

Beth called during the chair project. "Mother, you are a martyr!" she exclaimed. She pointed out that I could easily buy assembled chairs and have them delivered. What she couldn't see was that Phil and I still needed and wanted to do things together. While I was on the phone, he inserted bolts in random holes, but I managed to help him straighten out the simple assembly. We were working on two chairs for the two of us to have on our beach. Was this controlling? I didn't think so. I just wasn't ready to give up.

On my golf morning Heidi called at seven thirty to say she'd pick Phil up in half an hour to take him to day care. Phil told me he wasn't going anywhere with Heidi. On plan, I left before Heidi arrived. From the car, I called her back on my cell phone, warning her, "Heidi, your dad is fiercely determined to stay in *his* house." I also called my good friend and longtime housekeeper, asking her to keep an eye on Phil while she was cleaning our house, to call me if she was worried, and to fix him a hot dog for lunch. After twenty-five years of helping us, she was no stranger to Phil. They liked each other.

Heidi came to the house and talked frankly with her dad, though she could not convince him to come with her to Stillwater. She spoke of his Alzheimer's disease and need to accept help from others. He waved her off. Not wanting to reward his uncooperative behavior, she did not invite him out to lunch. As it turned out, Phil never knew the house-keeper was watching over him. He fiddled around, causing himself no trouble and accepted her preparing lunch. A new helping arrangement was born. The housekeeper extended her hours on Tuesdays, and day care went by the wayside. My one rule was that if she ever felt herself in danger, she should leave the property immediately and call me.

Phil had a new problem, however. He was beginning to be incon-tinent. I bought him new summer pants with bigger waists for easier unfastening. I allowed extra time in getting ready for bed or going out so that he would use the bathroom proactively. Still, in the morning wearing only his boxers, he often could not make the toilet, wetting himself, the floor, and the rugs in his path. At first he allowed me to steer him into the shower for an easy cleanup.

In a matter of weeks, Phil was having accidents during the day. Some times he noticed; other times he did not. He stank. I couldn't very well allow him to walk around soiled. Getting him to trade in his clothes and use a warm washcloth was not easy. Personal help was an art that I could not always effect with grace. In frustration, he began to push me away.

I was reminded of the horrific time years before when I had watched him disappear. One late winter afternoon when we were in our fif-ties, Phil and I had set out on a river walk with his hunting dogs. We often enjoyed the river in snow cover and quiet repose. No one else was around. The dogs drank thirstily from open seams of water at the river's edge. I suggested we stay on the beach for our walk, but Phil insisted the ice was safe. Out he went. I did not. Our parallel paths headed south toward the marina.

About twenty feet from shore, in front of the Homers' vacant lot, Phil plunged through the ice. In the flash of his disappearance, time stood still. I could see no lights on in the neighboring houses. The white expanse of treeless beach and broad river accentuated that I was alone in the vast landscape.

When Phil's head popped up, I took off my coat, thinking I had six feet of fabric from cuff to cuff to try to reach him. Terrified, my mind became very rational. I didn't want to get too close to the hole; I was quite sure that I did not want to go through the ice, too. It occurred to me that if we both drowned, our children would be orphans. Before I even ventured onto the ice, Phil—with Herculean strength and God's grace—managed to get his boot on top of the ice behind him, straighten his body, and roll free of the hole with adrenalin pumping.

"Why didn't you come out to help me?" he screamed.

I was shaking and speechless, trying in vain to strip him out of his heavy, wet coat so he could put on mine. He rebuffed such trifling help. I joined him in rage and stomped home, less than a quarter mile along the road. He followed—not his usual position.

At home, I did help him out of his nearly frozen clothes; encased, he could scarcely bend. Our tempers melted. When Chris returned home later, Phil told him about falling through the ice. It was then I heard Phil admit how close he'd come to losing his life.

In the middle of that night, I was awake and back in the kitchen, overwhelmed by loss and culpability. I faced the truth: I was unwilling to give my life in an attempt to save Phil. Over the years, I thought I'd done my best to help him past small and large mistakes, poor judgment, and occasional bad luck. When the doghouse he was building collapsed for lack of a building design, I had held it together until he could collect reinforcing materials. When he invested in Market House without assuring some limits on his liability, I was forced to help bail him out. Maybe I had to see that saving Phil was not my job. Self-preservation felt both acutely necessary and awful. Knowing that I could not or would not save him really shook me up.

The next morning I told Phil of my sleepless night. He was in his usual haste to get to the hospital for surgery. Having a real conversation was impossible. All he could say was, "I would have tried to save you without thought for my own life." As he hurried away, I knew he believed that to be true. When I arrived at my office at the bank, I set aside my work and wrote a spare piece entitled "Thin Ice."

| | |
|---|---|
| You | Me |
| Out you go | Not me |
| Falling through | Trouble |
| Saving self? | Drowned? Heart attack? |
| Help from shore? | What can I do? |
| Gone | No branch, my coat |
| Bobbing | Fear |
| Sliding, rolling, crawling | Relief |
| Stepping, dripping, shivering | Anger |
| On shore | Accused |
| Anger | Walking away |
| Home | Home |
| Melting | Helping |
| Silence | Numb |
| Confession | Listening |
| No joke | Truth |
| Reality | Exhaustion |

Heartsick from nearly losing him and from his quick step past the profound nature of the event, I had felt the icy water of loneliness close over me.

Now Phil was always on thin ice. His descents had to be chilling for him; they were certainly alarming to me. Knowing I could not save him, I was forced to watch him flounder. It was painful. My help was inadequate. At night, after Phil would fall asleep, I often sat alone in the quiet darkness, feeling swallowed by Alzheimer's shadow.

# CHAPTER 9

# Making the Decision

"Just do it," Dr. Holm said. "Phil needs a wife again." He knew that the pressures of full-time caregiving had all but erased Phil's and my feelings of being husband and wife.

Earlier in the spring, the children and I had listened to Wayne Caron outline the potential benefits of residential care. "Reframe the problem. Think what is best for Phil," he had told us. None of us had objected to the idea in what was an intellectual exercise. The closer we got to the prospect, however, the sadder I became. I didn't want to force Phil out of his home.

To me, our home was so much more than place, building, and address. It was where Phil belonged, where he was known and loved, where he was safe, where he could be himself. He had loved being a river rat, living along the St. Croix. Nature welcomed his tinkering. Planting trees and cutting down others, he worked the land with pleasure and expelled his stress in sweat. Known as the Pyro of the Point, he took refuge at his fire pit. Reducing debris to embers, stirring them until they turned to dust, Phil had sent smoke aloft for thirty-three years, a signal that he was happily at work with a dog at his side.

For the last three years we'd accommodated Alzheimer's, continuing to work together outside. Now, in the summer of 2006, I hired a landscaping service to bulldoze our large burning pit and plant grass seed. Bordered by cedar trees on one side, the large clearing opened onto fields of prairie grass and wildflowers. Phil and I were gladly transforming this space into a sanctuary for the August wedding of our neighbors' son. Our Chris and the young man had grown up together. We were delighted to contribute to his special day.

Phil spent contented hours in the shade nipping small twigs from the low branches of surrounding trees. Keeping an eye on him, I connected long hoses and moved sprinklers regularly from section to section. The landscapers installed pink roses along the gardening shed. Our work and the greening of the sanctuary carpet gave us natural togetherness and momentary, sweet reward.

I knew we were in serious trouble, though. Incontinence was raging. Phil didn't understand his problem. If he caught a whiff, he thought he'd stepped in dog poop in the yard. Changing his clothes did not occur to him. I could not tolerate him sitting down for lunch in his own excrement. Offering my help in cleaning up only added to his resistance.

Chris came home for the Fourth of July holiday. We always walked the mile into Afton for the annual parade. Phil got dressed before I convinced him to shower. I didn't get him to sit on the pot either, so he had a mishap. I stepped in his puddle in the back hall, turning my sock yellow. It was a showstopper. I asked Phil to come with me to our room for a moment and signaled Chris to disappear while I tended to the problem. Luckily, Phil cooperated in changing his clothes and washing up. (That had not been the case the day before.) When we reappeared, there was no embarrassment. "Ready, Dad?" Chris asked. "Go ahead, you two. I'll catch up in a minute," I encouraged.

I stayed to clean up the bathroom and back hall. The pail, disinfectant, and I were becoming good friends. Afterwards, I couldn't find my sunglasses, but I raced out the door anyway. When I caught up with the men, Phil was wearing my prescription sunglasses. I gently teased him and took the glasses. "Where are mine?" he asked. "Under your hat," I guessed. His glasses usually rested in his hat ready for all departures. He had in fact picked them up as a unit and placed them on his head. Chris watched this exchange with some amusement. Phil put on his own sunglasses, and we proceeded down the bike path to Afton.

After the holiday, Phil and I returned to our sanctuary project. Watching Phil and pulling the sprinkler to a new spot without looking where I was going, I walked full force into a thirty-foot-tall cedar tree.

Set firmly in place like an intractable problem, the tree trunk almost knocked me out. I fell to my knees and crumpled to the ground. I was painfully reminded once again that finding ways for us to work together could not erase the firm truth of his lousy disease.

I knew it was time to make changes. The idea of moving Phil into memory care assisted living frightened me. I anticipated and felt Phil's terror and anger. I didn't know if I could muster the courage to do it. My promise at diagnosis that we would be a team was in jeopardy.

In *Bird by Bird*, Anne Lamott writes of her discomfort in visiting a nursing home as part of her church's outreach. Initially, all she can see is broken people lined up like "wrecked cars." Eventually, a monk helps her see the residents as "trees in winter," still beautiful and deserving of unconditional love. I despaired of Phil's becoming a wrecked car or a tree in winter. At age sixty-six, he was too young! I was too young. I didn't want to lose him.

I lied about playing golf on Tuesday morning and went to see Wayne Caron. I was sporting an enormous black eye, a result of my collision with the tree. Assured that Phil had not decked me, Wayne gave me some toileting tips and encouraged initiating a search of memory care assisted living facilities. I didn't have the stamina to persist with the tips simply, confidently, and sweetly. I wanted to scream. At Heidi's urging, I finally removed the boxers from Phil's drawer and instituted Depends. Wayne had suggested avoiding this step if possible.

The paper briefs were a change, the very thing that confused Phil. I was awkward in helping him get into them. He didn't understand what the contraptions were for. Once on, they helped absorb and contain his waste. But he hated when they became heavy. Removing them was another issue. The pull-ups required removing his khakis too, which required removing his shoes. Nothing was easy. In frustration, Phil threw wet clumps of his used Depends around the bathroom. Failing to help him was literally shitty.

The next Tuesday I skipped golf again and visited memory care units while the housekeeper kept watch. I made up stories about my game and news of the other players for Phil while I secretly weighed options. My necessary investigation and duplicity betrayed his trust. Worse yet, many residents' bent figures and blank faces forced me to see our unwanted future. My strong, handsome husband did not yet look like these frail, impaired folks. I was heartsick.

Our children and friends supported the idea of placement, but I was the one who had to make the decision. I felt like a scared kid covered in goose bumps standing on a high dive. I needed to hold my nose and summon the courage to jump. I knew I couldn't live at the end of the proverbial diving board—neither could Phil.

That Saturday's support group at the university focused on different approaches and experiences that caregivers had had in placing their loved ones. Only one other member had done it without a lot of effort to soften the landing. "I knew my husband would not accept the option in advance," she sighed. Their doctor had been the responsible party for the decision, which the family implemented. That would have to be our plan. "Dr. Holm has prescribed a rest" would be my explanation to Phil if I got him there.

At my wit's end, I thought of one more possible source of help. A friend had sent me a book by Anne and Bob Simpson, *Through the Wilderness of Alzheimer's*. Anne was a friend of a friend. They both lived in northern Minnesota when the book came out, so I had not met Anne. Bob, a retired pastor, was in early-stage dementia at the time of the writing. As I read the book aloud to Phil in 2005, their two voices reinforced for us the value of marital relationship, dignity, and love. The disease had not erased the Simpsons' relationship nor taken away Bob's personhood. At least it had not at the point of publication. Their words allowed Phil and me to talk a bit about the difficulties we were experiencing. Such talking was rough terrain for us, but the exchanges had usually ended with hugs of assurance.

After their book was published, Anne and Bob had moved from Duluth to St. Paul because of his deteriorating condition and need for specialized care. My old friend wanted to introduce Anne and me personally, but it had not readily happened with her living out of town, Anne sorting new care alternatives, and me caregiving at home. Now with Phil needing residential care, Anne's name came to mind. I called information, got her home phone number, called her, and introduced myself.

She agreed to meet me for an early supper. We talked for four hours! I don't remember how I got away from Phil for this blessed meeting. Anne had placed Bob at Wellstead in Rogers, Minnesota, where he was—at least—safe. I had toured Wellstead on one of my "golf" days. Anne and I shared our heartaches. For me, she was a vision of loving perseverance and gentle strength. She radiated a hope that I needed. Perhaps I could do the unthinkable and still maintain a loving relationship.

Fortunately Wellstead had a place for Phil immediately. The director assured me that her staff was accustomed to handling difficult behaviors and seeing beyond them to the person. The facility had a favorable staffing ratio, but I couldn't help thinking that Phil was used to one-on-one attention. I longed to prepare him for the move without knowing how. "What if he explodes and ends up at Bethesda Hospital for behavior modification?" I stewed. I argued with myself, "We'll get through that if we have to." I tried to remember that the root of his upset was Alzheimer's, not me.

Dr. Holm told me that I gave Phil more credit for understanding than he had at that point. He made a one-time statement to Phil that he was directing us to Wellstead for help. As Dr. Holm predicted, Phil didn't register the significance of those life-changing words. In effect, the doctor's orders gave me permission and responsibility to admit Phil to a memory care assisted living unit. Fifty-two miles away, on the opposite side of the Twin Cities, Wellstead would have a new resident.

Heidi and I worked together to prepare Phil's room in advance. Wellstead provided a bed, a wardrobe, a nightstand, and a chair. I duplicated Phil's goose-necked, Verilux reading lamp and Bose radio-CD player. I chose his favorite CDs from our collection: big-band music, Dave Brubeck, Frank Sinatra, Tony Bennett, and Garrison Keillor's *Prairie Home Companion* anniversary set. While Phil was sleeping, I packed his preferred cotton slacks, golf shirts, a sweater, undershirts, tennis shoes and socks, a bathrobe, and toiletries. I stowed everything in the car trunk. On my next fictitious golf outing, Heidi and I drove out to Rogers. We stopped at Target to buy a few room accessories, laundry basket, and bulletin board. We spontaneously picked up a small desk and chair and limited office supplies. Punching in the code to unlock the courtyard gate, we couldn't look at each other. Lugging the stuff inside, I told her, "You hang up the clothes. I'll set up the Bose player." "Oh, Mom," Heidi groaned. We were almost robotic in tackling these practical matters, pushing down our feelings.

One resident wandered into Phil's room to watch the unpacking. We smiled at her, and she wandered away. I wondered how Phil would relate to these strangers and the quiet atmosphere. At least he would not have to negotiate hallways, as his room opened onto the dining area, where a row of windows looked out into the courtyard. The sunny day brightened the space as if to counter our gloom.

Meanwhile, Phil was clueless to our whereabouts. That night he and I had a chance to hear Dave Brubeck in concert. Not a musician himself, Phil was definitely tuned to music. As a child he'd enjoyed his parents' parties, which often included singing around the piano. He'd collected big-band records. In high school, he and a buddy discovered Brubeck on their own, going to outdoor gigs at the Walker. They even ventured to California in a souped-up station wagon to Brubeck's door. Mr. Brubeck wasn't home, but the boys nonetheless felt they'd arrived at the Source.

Over the years jazz had a way of transporting Phil and me out of the ordinary clutter of our lives. We used to create a night out by ourselves without all the familiar St. Paul faces paying proper and knowledgeable attention to the St. Paul Chamber Orchestra. Phil had predictably fallen asleep during those sedate concerts. Jazz worked better for us. We enjoyed the informality of small groups of musicians in the intimate setting of the Dakota. A set-side table with a light supper and a drink made us part of their action. We often did not know the performers, but they rewarded us with soulful riffs, taking turns in the spotlight and creating music as they went. We would hold hands and ride along. Drawn into the music, we felt their creative impulses and surprise outcomes as they glistened in sweaty effort.

Now, nearly five decades after discovering Brubeck, Phil had the opportunity to thrill to a live performance by the renowned musician. Could we leave Alzheimer's sitting in the lobby during the show? First we had to get ready to go. Buoyed by enthusiasm for the event and my patient help, Phil got into the shower, into his Depends, into his clothes, and into the car. The concert was magical. He tapped out the five-four rhythm on his knee and grinned like a Cheshire cat. Witnessing his swell of pleasure delighted me as much as the music itself. I did not think about Alzheimer's and Phil's leaving me. I savored our moment together.

Only a few days later, on August 9, 2006, Heidi and I had a different outing planned. Unbeknownst to Phil, we were taking him to Wellstead. The night before the move, I could not sleep. Getting ready for bed, Phil's disposable brief had fallen down as I removed his khakis. He didn't know what to do, except to demand privacy for his penis. He pushed me and tried to kick me. I stood my ground, telling him, "Phil, no rough stuff!" I turned around to throw away the Depends, and he jumped into bed bare-bottomed without using the toilet. I reapproached, asking him to use the toilet. He refused, glaring daggers at me. His despair was an odd blessing to help us toward separation. It was all too apparent that I could not help him in these delicate matters. He was truly angry with me. Strangely, I was not choked up. I just felt the weight of the inevitable. I felt like a used Depends myself.

The next morning, unperturbed by the previous night's struggle, Phil was pleased to go for a drive with Heidi and me. On the long ride we listened to music and acknowledged the sights out the window. Phil was not agitated, but we were. As we approached the facility, I piped up, "There is Wellstead, the place Dr. Holm told us about. Let's stop in and see what it's like." Phil was neither enthusiastic nor resistant. The three of us approached the building on a planned path into the sunroom. A friendly nurse was waiting for us. We all sat down supposedly to learn something about the place. Phil tried to participate in the conversation and agreed to see a unit where residents lived. When he saw his name on one of the room doors, he went ballistic. It was a locked unit, so none of us could get out. I admitted that Dr. Holm had prescribed his staying for a while "to rest his brain." There was no placating him. As an attendant distracted him, Heidi and I escaped with the help of other staff. The heavy door clicked shut, and Heidi sobbed in my arms. Our ruse had worked. The deceit felt dreadful. Any relief remained to be seen.

None of us had any idea what would happen next.

# CHAPTER 10

# Staying Afloat

'm going to kill you," he shouted at me. With coached calm, I looked him in the eye and said, "Phil, I can't stay if I upset you."

I was flanked by his cherished dogs. I hoped their presence would soften Phil's anger at having spent his first night in memory care assisted living. The dogs strained at their leashes, trying to reach him. I stood fixed, wary of advancing into his hot rage. He grabbed his belongings and deposited them by the door. His mind was racing, trying to escape his involuntary confinement. As confused as he was, he rightly targeted me as the one who put him there and could get him out. My heart pounded. The attempt to divert him with his much loved dogs was not working.

I waited two days and tried again. I knew not to sit in his room. Trapped in that dead end, I had suffered his physical and verbal threats on my first visit. I had barely managed to escape his room and exit the unit after a half hour. This time I asked, "Phil, will you sit with me at this sunny table? I would really like to be together." I struggled to keep my voice calm and my eyes on him. I hoped to connect, not incite. I knew Alzheimer's made conversation hard, but I wanted him to join me physically. He sat but soon demanded, "Let's get out of here!" I repeated the tired message that I wanted to be with him, but that I could not take him home now. His outrage forced me to leave abruptly again, without any hug of assurance. Staff suggested I stay away for awhile.

I called the unit daily to see how Phil was doing. I ached for him. The battle over clothing, toileting, and washing had resulted in staff injury on two occasions. Phil's violent resistance to personal care required more staff to come from other units. It reportedly took six helpers to get him into the shower.

Dr. Holm prescribed medication to help Phil with his extreme anxiety. Wellstead's management moved him to their all-male unit, where some of the certified medical assistants were men. I prayed that more camaraderie and fewer bathroom fights might result. For my own support, I went to see Wayne Caron.

Wayne affirmed that Phil's new antipsychotic drugs would slow down his racing mind and help stabilize his mood, but he also warned me that they might reduce Phil's functioning. "Barbara, as Phil loses function, his unhappiness will escalate. The medication might speed a downward spiral." So I added medications to my list of worries. Wayne reminded me that I was the most important person in Phil's life and that carrying that emotional support forward would be a challenge. Phil's threats, demands, and pleas showed that he was actually coping pretty well, according to Wayne. I continued to feel as though I was in free fall from that high dive, blown wildly by blasts of wind and with no landing in sight.

I had to trust Dr. Holm and the behavior reports of Wellstead staff. I didn't want Phil to hurt himself or others. I called the new unit for daily updates. Phil was beginning to accept personal care by the experienced staff. The unit leader told me, "Phil spends a lot of time in his room." I asked if he were sleeping during the day. The response, "I don't think so," did not comfort me. It seemed staff tended Phil, but they didn't always know what he was up to.

I called Dr. Holm for reassurance. He restated his therapeutic goal: "I'm trying to preserve and perhaps enhance Phil's functioning." The modest doses of medication were aimed at getting rid of Phil's rage and stabilizing his mood.

Dr. Holm thought it was a good idea for family to visit Phil to see if he appeared to be himself. Wayne thought Heidi and I should stay away in the near term so that we would not be retraumatized. The Wellstead director did not want me to come. The compromise was that Heidi's compassionate husband would go and report back to us on Phil's well-being. Phil was pleasantly surprised to see Rob. They went for a walk and talked about Rob's upcoming fishing trip with the grandchildren. Hearing about their normal exchange was such a relief!

The next day I willed myself to comply with the director's wishes for me to stay away, but my calls to the unit revealed that Phil was resting each time. That was not like him. The accumulated medications had kicked in. On Monday, twelve days after I dropped him off, I called the director. She was on vacation for a week. I gave myself permission to resume visits.

Phil was snowed. He was glad to see me and allowed lots of hugs, but he was in slow motion with vacant eyes. Independently, Wellstead staff and I called Dr. Holm to report this change. He discontinued one medication and reduced another. On my new daily visits I expected to see Phil immediately brighter and did not. I had to rouse him before lunch. He was droopy at the table and sleepy afterwards.

Several days later I took heart when Phil was not spent from the outset of my visit. Another day my visit coincided with a sing-along in the sunroom. Phil escorted me there; we held hands. He tapped his toe, clapped, and laughed appreciatively with the performers. Seeing him enjoying himself was a minor miracle. He joined in with no hint of concern for where he was, why he was there, or how long he had to stay. In that moment I believed our life together had been given back to us. I was Phil's wife again.

Chris called to check in. "What's going on, Mom?" Glad to hear his dad's mood was better and the meds less overwhelming, he asked, "So how are you doing?" In the two and a half weeks since Phil's placement at Wellstead, I had had real free time for the first time in years. Certainly the transition was tough on me as well as Phil. The first week was devastating. I could not move a pen to write in my journal, which ordinarily gave me pleasure. I felt like a bag of cement, mindless and inert. Sorting the seemingly conflicting messages of the professionals was hard work.

The good news was that I slept. I was very tired, and sleep came easily. Instituting daily visits to Phil after my initial banishment, I was developing a new rhythm; 24/7 care was over. Comparably, the long drive, the visit, and the necessary phone calls were a breeze.

In the interval, I had turned sixty-four. Heidi had a birthday party for me with family and friends. Everyone asked me in so many words, "Don't you feel cheated to be without your partner?" I hadn't really gotten to that question myself. I wasn't depressed as much as worn out. In my new free time, I pushed myself to be social. I kept thinking how much Phil was missing. He didn't know about my birthday or the neighbor's wedding in our yard; he couldn't feel left out of those festivities. Still, he was awfully far away from family and friends. I felt sort of split in half, trying to lead my own life as well as live our fragile peace.

Beth was in town. She baked Phil chocolate chip cookies and went with me to see her dad. He recognized her right away and happily settled at a patio table for the treat. He was neatly dressed. His eyes were clear. Beth complimented him on his sharp appearance. We all went for a walk on the grounds. Phil delivered a running commentary on the bushes, the flowers, the rocks, the bugs. In the end, he accepted that Beth had to go home to check on her babies, but he didn't understand that he could not go home with me. Clear of his drug-induced fog, he was able to reassert his plan to leave at once.

I was back in the position of reiterating that Dr. Holm had given orders for his "quiet time." I promised I'd be back the next day. Phil was annoyed. I kissed him good-bye and walked out. Before leaving the building, I asked the nurse to see him and evaluate any agitation. I called when I got home and learned that Phil had gotten over my departure, eaten his supper, and was waiting with the guys for the Twins game to start on TV. Within an hour, a Wellstead staff person called me: "Phil wants to speak to you." He insisted that I return immediately to get him. I listened and repeated that I would be there in the morning. I called the staff back an hour later. Phil was calm, watching the ball game. Phil probably didn't know the difference between immediately and morning, but inside I fought guilt that I had abandoned him.

I dreamed Phil and I were on a boat, searching for a mooring. Drawing close to a dock, I saw no cleat to tie up to. Cruising on, I discovered the craft had no lines with which to secure any dockage. Adrift, we had lost all ordinary means of securing connection. Popping awake, I tried to accept the reality of Phil's and my strange, new existence.

A month after Phil moved into memory care assisted living, we had a care conference. Wayne came out to Wellstead to participate. Confirming his attendance, I detailed the miracle of Phil's relative ease. "I'm really proud of Phil," he said. Indeed, my husband had done an amazing job of finding his way within his new environment. Wayne asked me what I wanted out of the meeting. I emotionally blurted out, "I want to feel that the staff know Phil, that they like him, that they think he's doing well, and that they are glad he is there." I'd also written a short list of more medical questions for the meeting, like "Has staff done an assessment of Phil?" and "What stage of Alzheimer's is he in?" I had thought when we signed up for Wellstead that there would be more activities for Phil to participate in. I needed to know why there were not more things for Phil to do.

Wayne was satisfied with the meeting. He thought we were fortunate to have such high-quality care. I took some assurance from this, but I couldn't help wanting even more for Phil.

At the end of September I left town for a two-day retreat with dear women friends. I was slightly tentative approaching the trip because I didn't know how I would handle the intensity of the group. Part of me hungered for real alone time to find my bearings and reenergize. As it turned out, the peer gathering was just what I needed. I relaxed into the moment. As I answered many questions about our Alzheimer's journey, I spoke from my point of view, from my wilderness experience, from my decisions, rather than just describing Phil's decline. Trading in honesty felt good. Others' interest and compassion felt good. I wasn't the only one with an agonizing story. We stayed in our pajamas until three in the afternoon telling our stories. Friends for fifty years, we laughed too, lightening up the mood with memories of our worst dates.

While I was gone, Heidi's family took Phil by car to a nearby sporting goods store for an hour. They peered into tanks of Minnesota fish and studied the many wildlife mounts. An avid hunter and fisherman, Phil was in his element. "Look at this, Grandpa," was a perfect invitation. After he devoured a juicy hamburger and onion rings in the in-store restaurant, Heidi alone returned Phil to Wellstead. She took time to settle her dad gently and quietly. It was a huge success.

Following Heidi's example, I eventually dared to take Phil on a different off-campus adventure. He and I took Sunny on a rather long walk to the Dairy Queen in Rogers. Phil enjoyed sharing his cone with Sunny. On the way back, I extended our route to a duck pond across the street from Wellstead. We watched dozens of geese on the water before climbing the hill to Phil's courtyard to check on the bird feeders I had installed. Phil was happy and full of smooches. Back inside, he took private time on the pot. I was hopeful that the pleasure of the activities and the relief of being cleaned up would put him at ease for my departure. Instead, Phil became tearful.

He'd long ago lost his ability to trade in accurate information, but he could still show his emotions. He was so soulful in wanting to go home. He told me, "I've been here for three years. I want my life back." He even wondered if he'd done something wrong that meant he had to stay there. I hugged him and rocked him. I whispered, "Oh, Phil, you have done everything so well, but the doctor has prescribed this quiet time." "Get rid of him," he countered. I could tell him I loved him. I couldn't tell him I could not take care of him by myself.

Just the day before I had emailed a large group of our friends, recounting a positive picture of Phil's adjustment. Both the story in my email and his angst were true.

Predicting his ease was impossible, however. One morning Phil and I returned from a walk outside and encountered another resident's spouse playing the piano in the sunroom. He was playing familiar, romantic tunes from the *Reader's Digest Family Song Book*, while an attendant walked his wife around the room. I asked the husband if we might listen for a while; he was glad to have us. "Phil, would you like to dance?" I smiled. In gallant fashion he bowed and then raised his arms in welcome. He led us in his usual graceful twirls and dips.

The pianist was having fun watching us. He kept playing. A half hour passed. We were all elevated and united in the music. Phil leaned into me and whispered, "We should make more babies." "Oh," I said, perhaps too literally but with tenderness, "aren't we lucky to have four babies already plus our eight grandbabies?"

Our unexpected dancing was such a kiss of grace. I had not felt abandoned by God in our difficulties, but that morning I was keenly aware of God's presence in our lives. That presence did not discount the pain of our circumstance. It did, however, illuminate the beauty in our relationship.

On my frequent trips to Rogers, I regularly passed the Silver Lake Road exit, leading to United Theological Seminary. I had enjoyed classes there before Phil's retirement. I thought about going back. I checked the seminary website and chose a writing class, Spirit and the Page. One session involved writing lists. I'd been good at making lists, particularly enjoying the crossing-off part. I was a doer who liked to be done. Straightforward grocery lists, places I wanted to go, things I wished to accomplish, people I needed to contact—this was the fodder of everyday living. In the class, listing my dreams and values was no problem. But the pen went dry, my hand went limp, and my mind went blank given the assignment to list my losses. I couldn't do it. I didn't see myself as a loser.

After class, I drove toward Phil and unintentionally exited prematurely. Perkins and pancakes beckoned. I sat down alone and stared at my spiral notebook that displayed only two losses: my loving father, who passed away at age ninety-two, and my childhood boyfriend, who had left me for a life abroad. Actually, I'd been fortunate: Dad's long life was a blessing in the family, and my first love affair was honest and sweet. My cell phone rang. It was Beth, who asked, "What are you up to?" I admitted that I was eating pancakes and trying to add to my list of losses. We laughed.

As days went on, my discomfort and inability to name loss weighed on me. I told my dear friend Abby about feeling derailed. Tangled emotions seemed to strangle my perception and hide words from me. I knew I'd skipped over my own feelings sometimes in trying desperately to find Phil some ease. I was in the midst of so much personal loss that I couldn't name it. I had been busy surviving. Abby suggested, "You are probably protecting yourself." I thought about it. My explanation was that the loss created by Alzheimer's was so big and close that my nose was against its hide. I couldn't even see the animal.

At the same time, after four months of Phil's stay at Wellstead, I was not merely feeling relief, I was experiencing an inexplicable sensation of glee. For sure, I was relieved to have Phil in a safe place with caring people to help look after him. But I questioned my joy in being able to take my leave from him. I even sought counseling to make sense of it. I came to accept that my decision to place Phil in residential care did not spring from some dark, unknown corner of my heart, but rather from my need to have some freedom myself. Alzheimer's had not only stolen Phil's insight and ability to care for himself but also imprisoned me.

From the beginning I believed that the decision to place Phil was right. Still, I was stunned by the fact of how much better I felt. I was enjoying being Phil's wife again. I was glad to be with him, to smile at him, to listen to him, to laugh together, even to weep together. His desires were uncomplicated: he wanted to be my man, my sweetheart, my love. My compassion and tenderness toward him grew as the rigors of my caregiving diminished. I was no longer operating on empty. By reclaiming some of myself, I had more to give to him.

# CHAPTER 11

# Speaking Out

With some free time after Phil's placement at Wellstead, I accepted an invitation to rejoin the board of the Amherst H. Wilder Foundation. I felt a bit awkward at first. I'd been gone for three years. The foundation was in the middle of a capital campaign for a new headquarters. Phil's residential care was expensive, but I wanted to plan a capital gift from our family. As I looked at the drawings, the building's backyard garden caught my imagination.

The cost of the backyard exceeded my means, but my imagination didn't give up. What if Abby and I did it together? What if the Dawkins and Roy families made the gift? Abby was like a sister to me, and Ken was my financial advisor; they loved me and admired Wilder. Abby had actually begun her social work career at Wilder.

I floated the idea, knowing Abby and I both valued the serenity of our own backyards. Phil's and my spacious land in the St. Croix Valley is where my thirst for natural beauty and the idea of stewardship really awakened. Settled in my native prairie, I felt so at home amid the waving grasses and sprinkling of wildflowers. The natural abundance comforted me.

Abby lived in the city, where her small yard was just as important to her as mine was to me. She knew the names of her flowers, neatly set in carefully planned beds. She knew what would bloom first and how to pinch spent blossoms to enhance more growth. She liked variety. She had some plants from her father's former garden in Massachusetts.

Every year she tried new species as well. Neighbors marveled at the colorful display. As different as our settings were, their value and purpose were the same. Our gardens spoke to us, comforted us, refreshed us, brightened our spirits. Intuitively, I knew we would enjoy making a backyard garden happen for Wilder—for the employees, the clients, and the barren neighborhood.

Ken cautioned me, "Barbara, you are the head of the household now. No salary exists to cover living expenses. And you need to maintain financial flexibility to weather market downturns and family emergencies." True, but I still wanted to make the gift. I examined various sources of funds and considered pledging over a period of years. In the end, the two families made the gift together. I was thrilled for Wilder and for myself. Having time to think again without constant interruption and concern for Phil's needs was reinvigorating.

Chris came home for a visit. I told him happily about the return of my imagination and the proposed garden at Wilder. He was excited for me to be reclaiming some of my old life. We went together to pick up Phil so we could all go to the Saturday support group at the university. Afterwards, the three of us ate lunch at Muffaletta and walked around the Como Conservatory. Easy companionship, good food, and a nature activity suited all of us. Tom Kingston's name popped into Phil's mind. He told Chris, "He's a good man." I agreed, "He's a great leader at Wilder." On the drive back to Wellstead, I drove us by the Wilder construction site. I circled the area and told Phil simply, "We are making a contribution to the garden." I did not delve into why it meant so much to me. I hoped we could visit the garden together when it was finished.

Arriving back at Wellstead, Phil was surprised and angry, verbally refusing to go "back there." Nevertheless, I parked, suggested Dove Bars in the sunroom, and led us into the building. In spirit Phil was resistant, but in habit he followed along. The tension of return was part of the emotional price of our outings. It would have been easier to tell Chris over the phone, "I took Dad to Como today." I hated having him see the struggle of reentry, Phil's unhappiness, and my effort to complete the outing. Was I wishing to protect Chris or to run away from my fear that Phil's adjustment was not assured? Wayne Caron's accusation that I was "controlling" rang true. The glee that surprised me after placing Phil in residential care was definitely not a perpetual state of mind.

Knowing that I'd recently placed Phil in residential care, the head of Wilder Research asked me to be one of the speakers at a forum on elder needs and services held in February 2007. Wilder's Perspective Series typically featured professionals in a given field and presented relevant research. I wasn't qualified to give one of Wayne's scholarly presentations, but I could put a face on the role of caregiving. Going public with my experience was a bit daunting, but I knew public awareness of the caregiver role was important. Community decision makers at the forum might benefit from my personal story of needing and finding help.

What had I learned? I didn't want to recite the nitty-gritty details of our falling apart. I wasn't ready to talk about Phil as a case subject. I didn't want to sugarcoat my caregiving job with a notion of willing self-sacrifice. And even though memory care assisted living was working pretty well for us at the moment, I knew that its success was tenuous, not fully assured. Mulling what I might say, I settled on three lessons that I'd learned under fire.

I arrived promptly at the University of Minnesota for the unrehearsed forum. Putting on my speaker's badge, I felt like a poster child for Alzheimer's care. Two hundred people, nearly all of whom I didn't know, filled the auditorium. I was introduced as a Wilder Foundation board member who had personal caregiving experience. Representing the foundation, I wanted to be articulate and informative. Confident on the outside and shaking on the inside, I stepped to the podium.

I waited a moment, looking around the room before I began to speak. I admitted my reluctance in becoming a caregiver and offered my three lessons:

*First, no one can do this work alone.* At the same time, caretaking is so consuming that finding space to ask for help is not easy. "I am lucky. Our family and friends have given my husband and me huge emotional and practical support, but that does not change the reality that Alzheimer's disease has an intractable isolating effect. It's relentless, tiring, and unpredictable."

*Second, needs change, and new dilemmas arise. In other words no plan, however good it might be, lasts.* Continuous decisions must be faced.

Seeking a diagnosis is a big step, but many other steps ensue, like creating a power of attorney, reviewing finances, assessing the current living arrangement in terms of physical needs, determining what activities no longer make sense, accommodating the extra time needed to maintain the activities that still work, inviting family discussion, deciding what to tell friends and how to call on their help, lining up volunteer and/or professional services, and figuring out what community resources are available, affordable, and a good fit. "While I tended to these matters, I also had to recognize my personal limits and exhaustion. I needed to refuel and maintain a sense of humor."

*Third, in some ways the caregiving journey is heartening.* Despite all the changes in the loved one and all the necessary lifestyle adjustments, much remains precious. With life slowed down, there is time to hold hands. "When there's a lull in the lunch conversation, my husband cheerfully offers up, 'Hi ho, silver!' He performs his duck call to delight the grandchildren. He talks to their photographs. He swings me in a dance step. He reports the glad news to staff that he's seen his grandsons play hockey. He's no longer concerned about winning. His odd, layered costumes do not hide his smile. He seems to be about being himself in appreciative relation to others. I laugh at his antics. His goofiness delights others. I feel his essence untrammeled by oughts and musts. Despite our separate living arrangements, his confusion, and my own weariness, I feel close to him."

All of us in that room knew we did not want to be a burden on our spouse, our children, or society. I continued, "I am relating my personal story because our culture dreads frailty, incapacity, dependency. Most of us think that asking for or needing help would be painful, when in reality it can open hearts. Our family system is being tested and not found wanting. Both Phil and I are awed by our children's consideration and affection. Friends have been wonderfully thoughtful, steadfast, and creative on our behalf. The professionals we've encountered, who have chosen this field as physicians, psychologists, nurses, and aides, are remarkable folks. The other families we've met facing Alzheimer's disease model incredible courage. While I would never have chosen the Alzheimer's experience, I am nonetheless grateful for the beauty of these special people in our lives."

I concluded, "What I worry about for other families is the added pain of financial impossibility. We have had medical insurance and retirement savings that have allowed our decisions to be driven by what has been best for Phil. Without me available to care for my husband, he would have required professional care far sooner. Without our medical insurance and savings, we could not have crafted the plans we made. Working on our taxes for last year, I have identified over $50,000 in out-of-pocket care costs for 2006, which included only five months of memory care assisted living. That is a troubling number for any family, especially as the costs will grow annually and cease only with death. Minus the financial implications, caregiving alone consumes the emotional purse." I sat down.

Afterwards, people I didn't know hugged me. The people I did know thanked me. I hurried on my way to see Phil. Driving along, I wondered what Phil would have thought about my public story. I was glad that I'd stood up and been able to speak out, and I was well aware that our story was not over.

Two summers later, a professor at the University of St. Thomas in St. Paul asked Abby to lead a class on grief and loss. She invited me to do it with her. She remembered my blank response to the seminary exercise to list my losses. I agreed to dive inside myself and try again for words. I told her I would let her know. Phil had been in residential care almost three years by then. The relentless, ever-changing, heart-filled experience of living with chronic illness remained in full swing.

As I wrote, Phil's losses came easily to the page, and then mine did, too. I saw myself as a loser. I allowed the hurts and disappointments, the incremental agony of the deathless death over the seven years of Phil's decline. I laid myself bare, smelled the stench, and tasted the bitterness. I embraced my own vulnerability. These things had not been absent in my journal writing, but this time I didn't balance them with good news in my life. I let them pile up like dirty laundry: rumpled, stained, and unwearable. Writing gave me the chance to spill out the tough stuff knotted deep inside, to look at it squirming on the page, to cast aside the niceties.

My writing didn't match the excellence of John Bayley's *Elegy for Iris*, but it was my voice with our experience settled onto the page in full lament. Reading Bayley and Iris Murdoch's story had been poignant confirmation for me of the agonizing descent into Alzheimer's. Both brilliant academics—Bayley, an English literary critic, and Murdoch, a philosopher and novelist—they were practiced in solitary pursuits, much as Phil and I had been. The "closeness of closeness" caused by Alzheimer's was new territory in their marriage. Bayley warned me, "No point in getting away from it all, nowhere to get away to. Alzheimer's will meet you there, like death at Samarra." And he clarified for me, "Anger sometimes seems now to be a way of still refusing to admit that there is anything wrong. You are just the same as ever, bless you (or curse you), and so shall I be." Such powerful truths!

I decided to take the risk to collaborate with Abby at St. Thomas and share my truth with the graduate students pursuing degrees in social work. This time I was not representing the Wilder Foundation. Wearing jeans, I sat at a table in a small classroom of desks and introduced myself as a very positive person, one who always saw the glass half full. I hoped these students would see me as a potential client faced with the difficulty of caring for a husband with Alzheimer's.

I quickly described my denial early on, hardheaded pragmatism along the way, and tender attention to whatever remained in our relationship during Phil's descent. I wanted them to see how Alzheimer's stole our way of doing things and attacked both of us: Phil as the victim of illness and me as his wife and eventual caregiver. I ticked off the losses.

Phil's first loss was confidence, which meant he wanted to do everything together. My concurrent loss was personal freedom. I felt as if I were in a children's game of Captain, May I?, needing to request his permission for my every move. In my maturity, I wasn't used to explaining or asking permission for my whereabouts. Our togetherness became ever more necessary and smothering. Phil repeatedly asked, "What are we going to do now?" If I had a solo outing, he would complain, "You just saw So-and-So. What am I supposed to do?" His sense of time evaporated. My saying, "I'll be back in an hour," simply meant he would be alone. His need for companionship rose to the point where I simply could not leave him.

Phil lost his thinking powers, and I lost my ease. Numbers were an early problem for him; he could not tip at restaurants or calculate handicapped golf scores. Fortunately, he was pretty gracious about my taking over all financial matters, work that I was already good at. He trusted me; he certainly did not want to lose his money. Being mathematically challenged was a comeuppance for Phil, but not really dangerous. Unhappily, I became a detective, watching for other signs of trouble.

Phil lost his judgment, and I lost my partner I could count on. I considered one of the bonuses of marriage to be that husband and wife took up different responsibilities to make the unit run smoothly. On a mundane level, Phil was in charge of our dogs. He dutifully fed them; actually, he overfed them. The vet cautioned us to cut back their food. After Phil entered residential care, the dogs became my sole responsibility. I mustered the energy to take good care of them for Phil's sake. Sadly my affection for them began to dry up over time. I couldn't feel the joy they so willingly bestowed on Phil. Their faithfulness was lost on me. The need to care for them only added to my mounting despair that I was losing Phil. When Phil no longer drove, I became a full-time chauffeur. It would have been nice to have been driven sometimes. I'd enjoyed our former road trips when my turn as passenger had allowed me to watch the scenery or read the AAA guide about the area we were passing through. Putting my head back and relaxing were out of the question with Alzheimer's in the car.

Phil lost his organizing skills, and I lost orderliness in the house. He would discover special treasures in drawers and arrange them on counters for easy access or tuck them into unusual places, where they went missing. When possible, I redirected him to work in his garage shop. Without large power tools, he still had dozens of screwdrivers, hammers, boards, cans of paint—lots of stuff to work with. He covered the garage walls with odd board lengths and screwed red plastic creamer caps onto the heads of carved cardinals in our garden. He was both pleased and dedicated. I used those brief times of his independent endeavor to work at my desk to keep our affairs in order. I missed his help in washing the cars, trimming the trees, and making his secret recipe for salad dressing. His independent work no longer improved our life. I was lucky if it didn't disrupt it.

I paused before outlining the hardest part. When Phil lost empathy, I lost graceful connection. The marital relationship succumbed to a full-time caregiving relationship in which my authority was difficult for both of us. Phil's early gratefulness and my natural willingness to spend more and more time together tipped over with the weight of the growing responsibility that fell to me. He could not see that I had all that much to do, that I was tired, that I was lonely, that we were isolated. In scant private moments with our children, they were frank with me. They missed me and lovingly demanded to know how I was managing.

Despite my efforts to preserve Phil's dignity, he eventually came to see me as the problem. His losing continence busted our helping mode. My coaxing him to the toilet to prevent accidents was futile. He would shout, "I don't have to go to the bathroom." When accidents occurred, my gentle persuasion toward warm water, soap, and towels in the bathroom took forever. Changing clothes had long before become a difficult, two-person task in which Phil had little interest. Showering was no longer a daily practice. Incontinence required both practices many times. I despaired of his circumstance and my inability to help him.

Residential care gave me some respite and Phil an easy routine, but it clearly did not change the fact of loss. Phil shrieked at me, "You cannot take away my home, my family, and my friends!" I was not the guilty party; Alzheimer's was. Still, the harsh reality that he was *not* at home with easy access to family and friends was crushing for both of us. Phil suffered an acute loss of belonging; I lost my precarious role of being in charge.

I smiled telling them Phil also lost his angst. One day when I entered the unit, he greeted me, "My queen is here." We planted pots of flowers and set up bird feeders. We were not without enterprise and even delight. To some degree we had each other back. Nevertheless, I lived alone and suffered a very long drive to see him.

Mostly, I told the class, I missed small things. Phil and I had already enjoyed enough big plans together to fill a lifetime. On the other hand, he could no longer bring me a cup of tea. We no longer read the paper together, calling attention to different articles. We no longer watched each other happily and guiltily slather butter on fresh corn. "Want to go for a walk?" and "Let's do a movie" could no longer be spontaneous invitations. Driving home from Phil's care center one evening, I'd tried a movie by myself. The dateless date was miserable—even the popcorn had tasted wrong.

I wanted the class to know that I did make and execute plans on my own. I had recently driven to the Black Hills to fish and hike with our son, Chris. South Dakota sunflowers saluted me along the highway; I was exhilarated to be on my way. Enjoying an adventure that Phil would have loved actually produced warm feelings. On my drive back to Minnesota, I stopped for dinner all by myself. Waiting in the booth for the food to be served and staring at the empty, facing bench, I lost it. I wept for Phil, who had missed out on the trip. I wept for me, who had no one with whom to share the memory at that moment. I couldn't ask, "Didn't Chris look great?" or "Do you think Amber might be the one?"

At the end of the class I read a poem written by my wonderful new friend Anne Simpson. Recently Anne had been working on a cooperative exhibit with her photographer cousin, Laura Crosby. *I'm Still Here!: The Alzheimer's Story* featured Laura's pictures paired with Anne's poems. Laura's black-and-white photo of Phil watering his pansies in the care center's courtyard faced Anne's poem "Resurrection":

> We shed like dry leaves
> our beauty
> our health
> our loved ones
> the places we have belonged,
> all such stuff as we are made of.
>
> We wriggle our roots
> deep into the soil
> from which we came,
> to which we return.
>
> Our branches,
> gnarled and bare,
> stretch out to bless the world
> we cannot hold,
> reaching to the sky
> and waiting for spring.

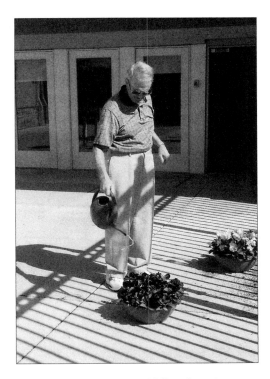

*Phil watering his pansies at Wellstead, 2007*

I told the students I found comfort in the belief that Phil would experience new life in death and resurrection. He need not and could not hold onto all the earthly things he was. When I no longer would be able to hold his hands, look into his blue eyes, comb his hair, or share his company, I imagined wishing him Godspeed to new life—not as a swashbuckling surgeon nor as a frail, crooked old man, but rather as a unique human spirit returned to the Divine.

Though I was accustomed to public speaking, coming out as a loser was new. I had opened up and allowed others to see inside. Exposing Phil's and my vulnerability inducted us both into the human family as losers. Some students wept; others asked questions. Their sincere responses encouraged warm dialogue. I began to see our truth as a gift I could give others.

# CHAPTER 12

# Overdoing

The first year I ever lived independently was 2007. Married two weeks after graduating from college, I had lived with Phil for forty-three years. Now I had our whole house to myself and time to design my new life, or so I thought.

I was drawn to Wellstead like a powerful magnet. My departures from Phil took resolve. Six months into his stay, he was growing angry again. He often clouded up when I said good-bye. One day he threw fistfuls of dog biscuits at me. The best I could do was to stay calm and continue on my way. After I left, he launched water bottles, like hand grenades, out of his room into the common area. Staff called to assure me he eventually settled down. Phil's erratic behavior exhausted both of us.

On the long drives back and forth to Rogers, I listened to *Moby Dick* on CDs. I enjoyed Melville's language and humor. I identified with Ahab and pictured the white whale as Alzheimer's. The whale would disappear for periods and then surface with fury. Ahab's maniacal pursuit ended with his harpoon sunk into the beast, the harpoon line around his own neck, and the beast pulling him to his death in the deep. Fortunately, unlike Ahab, I did have a sense of self-preservation. Phil's coiled anger drove me crazy, though. I knew Phil saw me as his lifeline. He didn't want to drown either.

I took him back to St. Paul to see Dr. Holm. Phil had forgotten that Dr. Holm had written the prescription for his stay at Wellstead. He was glad for an outing, cooperative with the nurse, and chatty with Dr. Holm. His chatter was scarcely on topic, however. He couldn't track my reporting or the medical advice. I reported a recent, unhappy exit in which Phil grabbed and shoved me, banged pitiably on the door I escaped through, and threw the common room furniture. Awakening the next morning, he had swung his putter around his own room and bashed the wardrobe. Dr. Holm made medication changes and wrote orders for Haldol PRN (as needed), the medication that calmed Phil in Texas.

Phil was furious when he saw that I was pulling back into the Wellstead parking lot. "We have to deliver Dr. Holm's papers," I told him. "You could have mailed them," he shot back. Where did that clear thinking come from? I was so confused. He made no sense most of the time. Once inside, my attempt to be pleasant went nowhere with him. I left. I had to get away.

I called Dr. Holm from the parking lot. He called the unit and told the nurse to administer the Haldol. I trusted Dr. Holm, but I also felt as if I were in a conspiracy to push Phil's head under water. Sadly I understood that nobody could care for Phil when he was full of rage.

After a week, the change in medication helped. Phil settled down. I took him out for an early supper. Mother happened to call my cell phone while we were eating. I put Phil on the line. "I've been taking care of a lot of seniors," he said and added that he hoped his speaking of seniors needing care did not upset her.

Phil's quarterly care conference took place several days later. Heidi, the Wellstead nurse, the executive director, and I faced each other at a small table in the director's office. The director gave a general summary of Phil's "behaviors," concentrating on the very upsetting ones that resulted in our meeting with Dr. Holm. She attributed Phil's manic and abusive behavior to being overstimulated and rather quickly came to her point. Looking at me, she said, "You do too much with Phil." She knew I was going out of town for a few days to see my mother in Texas. "Stay away for a week. Phil needs to reorient at Wellstead," she told me. She didn't want other family members or friends to come in my place. She didn't seem to be taking into account that the medication changes to counter Phil's "mixed-mood disorder" were helping. I was angry. "So, what do you think will be different, if we take your course?" I demanded. Heidi tried to soothe me, "Mom, let's just see how things go with the medication changes *and* no visits."

Jena met me in Texas to help celebrate Mother's ninety-fifth birthday. I was looking forward to seeing them. When I called Phil's unit to see how he was doing, staff told me, "Phil's okay, but he's having a hard time finding his room." He'd gone into another resident's room and pulled the poor fellow off his bed onto the floor. When a staff person came to check out the commotion, Phil told her, "He was on my bed!" I was grateful for her handling the matter without recriminations. No one was hurt.

Returning to Phil after a week's absence was sweet. His eyes were closed. I kissed his lips and told him he smelled good. Staff had convinced him to take a bath that morning. His eyes fluttered open. He smiled and whispered, "Barb?" He did not complain about my being gone; he just looked at me in seeming relief. I raised the blinds in his room on the beautiful day outside. He commented on the discarded, windblown, construction paper in the field across the street. "Let's go outside," I suggested. I helped him into his jacket and brought along a trash bag. We ended up collecting litter and hiking around the building to the dumpster. Phil had not lost his pleasure in helping. Inside, we washed up, and he told staff proudly what we'd been doing. They were glad to see us back together.

Dr. Holm wanted to see Phil for a follow-up. While we waited in the lobby of his hospital office, a nurse in the adjacent Capistrant Center for Parkinson's Disease, recognized Phil. "Dr. Roy, I used to work with you at Midway Hospital." Phil beamed. A conversation of sorts ensued. Dr. Holm found Phil "looking good," made no further medication changes, and gave us an appointment in three months. We were back on track.

My departures no longer raised alarm. Perhaps my activities to entertain Phil had been excessive. Perhaps his confidence that I was back gave him new peace. Perhaps the medication was in full effect, reducing his exaggerated feelings. Perhaps he was simply becoming more institutionalized. In any case, I knew I was relieved not to be cast as an escapee. Not battling separation had to be better for Phil, too. He was a bit slower, but his affect was bright and his tenderness genuine.

In May I went to San Francisco. Beth urged the plan and bought me the ticket. Her young family had moved there from New York City, and their newly remodeled house was ready for a guest. I did not tell Phil I was going. I used to think explanation and details grounded him in the truth, but now I understood that my telling only gave him something to worry about or confused him. Heidi visited in my absence. I imagined Phil tending the pots of pansies we'd bought for the courtyard. One of the residents, who rarely spoke, had said, "Pretty," when we'd carried them in. Phil's interests added a touch of excitement to a subdued atmosphere. He liked to show his flowers to the other residents.

At home I attempted spring cleanup in our yard. I missed my faithful helper. Even though Phil had mostly watched me the previous year, I had had his support. I nipped dried stalks and carted them to the refuse pile with a sense of loss. Without a prairie burn, I could identify the weeds because they were green. I wanted them eliminated. I finished one patch and turned around to find more. Also, I wanted to be on my way to Wellstead.

In June I went to New York City with my high school women friends to celebrate our sixty-fifth birthdays together. When I returned, Phil's older sister, Barbara, called with the sad news of her husband's death. Glad for my new flexibility, I rushed to Detroit. Of course Phil would have wanted me to go, but again he knew nothing of my travel. He mostly knew what he could see in concrete terms, and even then he got mixed up. He tried to drink the liquid candle at P. F. Chang's when I took him there for lunch.

The freedom to be with others in fun and in sorrow gave me new life. Travel also taxed my energy. I just kept going. At my invitation, Mother arrived for the summer. I'd missed her during Phil's long illness. His demanding home care had precluded her staying with me for years. She was excited to see my children, all of whom were also coming to visit during the course of the summer. We all were anxious to be together. And to add to the excitement, I lent my yard to a dear friend for her son's wedding. I barely knew how to pace myself! At the same time, I never forgot Phil in the swirling confusion. Thankfully he didn't have to live it day by day; he could never have tolerated it.

Heidi continuously knocked herself out trying to create doable events at their family's river house so Phil could participate. On Father's Day I picked him up early to drive back to the river by eleven. Rob and their son Walter, age eight, were fishing from the dock and immediately gave Phil a rod to hold. When Heidi served lunch, Susan, age six, suggested we go around the table and say something nice about the person sitting next to us. Phil couldn't offer anything except his smile. Next, Heidi announced a pontoon ride. Holding my hand, Phil gamely negotiated the dock, stepped aboard, and sat awkwardly confined in his life jacket. The wind had picked up. Every wave exaggerated his precarious position on the edge of the cushioned bench. The children whooped when the spray splashed them; Phil winced. Heidi could see that this fun was too much. She returned us to the dock. Phil was able to say, "It's time to go home." He didn't mean our house; he meant Wellstead.

When Jena's family came for the Fourth, Heidi repeated the family picnic at the river. I worried that Phil might become confused with so many of us. During the car ride I emphasized that we would get to see Jena and our grandchildren Max, age thirteen, and Mimi, age twelve. He looked momentarily puzzled seeing all the faces. Jena came forward, "Hi, Dad, it's Jen." He recognized her. When Mimi approached him, he responded with silliness. He definitely felt the family connection. We didn't overstay. That time, the pontoon ride occurred after our departure.

Beth's family was in town on his birthday on the ninth, and Heidi provided another gathering. It was deathly hot. Phil didn't understand his own birthday; he ignored the grandchildren's presents. He wouldn't sit down for the cake. The kids blew out the candles and enjoyed it themselves. The hardest part was that he paid no attention to Beth and her toddlers. Unlike Jena, she couldn't break away from her children to approach him by herself. Cait, not feeling well, clung to her mom, and Imogen required strict watching by the water. In the confusion Phil wandered the patio and muttered to himself. I thought maybe he needed to use the restroom, but that was unsuccessful as well. As I got him back into the car, Heidi sighed, "That was the worst!" Beth knew her dad was failing and might not recognize her, but experiencing the disconnect was grim.

Phil's adventures to the St. Croix were done. Of course, family members went to Wellstead to see him. His sister Barbara came from Detroit. Armed with Phil's favorite dark chocolate–covered cherries, she helped him open the box and together they popped the sweets into their mouths. In the courtyard, she deadheaded the pansies, I watered, and Phil wandered happily about talking to the air. She made us root beer floats. Phil allowed me to feed him spoonfuls. Finally, I turned on the Twins game and smooched him good-bye. "Thanks for the nice day, sweetheart." Keeping the family time in his setting with simple activity worked.

One day Mother went with me to see Phil. He greeted us enthusiastically and gladly went with us to nearby Maynard's for lunch. I ordered his usual halibut fingers and tartar sauce. During the meal he suddenly frowned and said something to the effect that he was not glad that he'd given away all his stuff. I wasn't sure what he was referring to. His tools? His house? Then it occurred to me that he might mean something in his room. "Don't worry, Phil, your things are probably in the laundry room," I said, hoping I could steer him away from real disappointment. He could have thought my response odd, but we moved on. Understanding his words and nonverbal communication was a growing challenge. On the other hand, I did not miss his all too clear expressions of anger.

Back at Wellstead, Phil popped out of the car and headed off, while Mother was still trying to get her legs under herself. With some corralling, I got both of them into the air-conditioned building. They both needed to use the bathroom. I left Mother to use the sunroom restroom and took Phil into his locked unit. His legs were rigid; he couldn't get himself to sit down. We gave up. Pants up, he collapsed into his lounge chair and closed his eyes. I put on soft music and kissed him good-bye. Mother was happily waiting in the ice cream parlor. She'd found a small carton of strawberry ice cream and a plastic spoon for the ride home. An accident, construction, and a stop for gas made the trip back last two hours. I was tired.

In September, Phil's sister Allie and stepmom, Sally, flew to Minnesota. They had not seen their beloved Phil since the Dallas blowout eighteen months earlier. Sally's mom and sister had suffered from

Alzheimer's, so she knew what to expect. Allie did not. At Maynard's, she watched her big brother dip his fruit into the tartar sauce. Savoring the memory of his kind touch, she gently took his slippery hand and told him, "Phil, you have the most wonderful hands." He accepted her tenderness.

We took Phil back, and Allie made it all the way outside before bursting into tears. "I don't know if I can go back tomorrow," she wailed. We did, of course. Phil had eaten his breakfast and was sitting in the common room when we arrived. We drew our chairs close to him to chat. He showed us the photograph of an ape he was holding. I retrieved his monkey portrait book from his room. The expressive monkey faces invited mimicry. Soon we were all laughing. Allie asked Phil to take her on a walk to the duck pond. He "led" the way, with me quickly unlocking doors and gates as they approached. He also showed her the indoor fish tank and ice cream parlor. When I finally announced that it was time for the airport, Phil did not protest. It was also time for his lunch. Much relieved, Allie told me in the car, "I'd never move him. What a great place!"

Revolving family staying in my house kept me company. Living with Phil had been lonely. Mother's visit was such a treat for both of us that I extended it through October. As much as she loved me, she did not like cold weather. Texas and Ted's ranch were her new home, but fall in Minnesota worked. Beth's family returned. After the little ones were asleep, Beth and Mother challenged me to nightly Scrabble games. Beth urged Mother, "Come on, Gram, we need to pull out our A game tonight!" Mother couldn't see the board clearly, but she happily partnered with Beth and helped form words on their rack. They always won. Beth's enthusiasm and silly competition pleased me, too.

Three-year-old Cait, quite like her mother, always wanted to know the plan for the day. "I'm going to see Grandpa," I explained. Her "me too" encouraged Beth to pack up her tribe for the journey to Wellstead with me. Phil needed to poop when we arrived. I took him to the bathroom, but nothing happened until we all stood before the fish tank. Cait said to Imogen, "You pooped!" Indignant, Imogen said to her, "You pooped!" I led Phil back to his room for cleanup. Beth and the girls played in the sunroom until we could return to blow bubbles. Phil was delighted by the children without really knowing who they were. But he also paid attention to Beth, who was touched.

A primary objective of Beth's trip to Minnesota was to baptize the girls in my meadow. Oliver's English uncles and Canadian parents joined us. Heidi's family decided to participate as well. My wonderful minister, who had married Heidi and Rob on our lawn fourteen years earlier, agreed to lead the service with Oliver's uncle John, a priest. It made no sense to include Phil physically. Instead we used a table that he'd made in his workshop as the altar and placed one of his bonsai trees on it. A glorious day blessed all of us as each child received the sacrament. Holding hands in the four-generation family circle, I felt God's gracious love. Afterwards, I served a simple dinner for eighteen.

Beth had another idea. Why not remodel Phil's workshop into a guest room? Certainly my place had been crowded, and another room and bath would have been handy. Mother chimed in, "I want to contribute. I take up one of the rooms. You don't have enough space for all your children." I studied the layout to determine how the workshop could be shut off from the garage and opened into the house. I called our old architect to draw a plan. Suddenly, I had a new project to complete by the time everyone returned for Christmas.

With an empty house in November, I dreamed I was taking an exam in law school. (I'd never been to law school.) I wasn't prepared as much as I would have liked, but I was comfortable enough with blue book and pen in hand. When I went to see the professor and discuss my exam results, she suggested to me that law school wasn't really for me. I was surprised. No one had ever directly told me that I couldn't do something. Not out of passion for the law but on principle, I objected, "I'm smart. I understand nuance." She handed me the exam. I'd failed.

At the time of the dream I couldn't make much of it. I woke up disheveled, unsure of myself, and flattened. I wrote it down in my journal with a question mark. In recollection, it's easy to see that I wasn't all that smart in dealing with Alzheimer's. Our Alzheimer's course was a failing proposition. Surely I had cared deeply. Mostly I had coped effectively. But definitely, I had overdone.

## CHAPTER 13

Examining Marriage

Marriages unravel. In our case, Alzheimer's was like a scissors snipping away at Phil's capacity to participate. Sadly, Jena's marriage was unraveling, too. I loved our oldest daughter; her husband was like a son to me. Their heartache went to my quick.

In late 2007, when I was on a visit to Boston, Jena asked me, "Mom, why did you stay married?" Over the years, there were times when I had imagined myself unbuckled from Phil and our marriage, times when I'd wanted to free myself from the unhappiness I felt, times when I had felt very stuck. Part of the answer, for me, was in accepting the struggle, neither ignoring it nor expecting a perfect resolution. Living the struggles, owning my pain, and accepting being human had allowed me to grow and helped Phil to grow as well. I'd shed tears and preconceived notions. Being "right" had been no more fun than being "wrong" for either of us.

I admitted to Jena that when Phil and I married, neither of us was comfortable expressing our feelings, especially feelings around our own vulnerabilities. I stated the obvious, "It's hard to listen if no one is talking." I remembered shouting at Phil once, "You make me sick!" That was a silence breaker for both of us. It might have been kinder to say, "I feel sick at heart; I feel alone even when we're together." Both statements were true, but the first one got his attention.

While in Boston visiting Jena's family, I went to Susan and John Gunderson's home for supper. Very old friends of Phil's and mine, they knew our children too. We sat by the fire to catch up. I confided that I was sad because Jena's marriage was in trouble. John, a highly respected psychiatrist at Harvard, studied me. "So, Barbara, what kind of example were you for Jena?" he asked. I was not offended. I'd asked myself the same question.

I said that Jena had left home for Dartmouth at age eighteen, before I'd effectively confronted Phil with my serious need for change in our marriage. Our standoff over the Market House investment was the visible tip of an iceberg. She had witnessed Phil's unreliable moods and behaviors that I did not call out in front of the children. I said, "I think Jena felt her dad was untrustworthy and I was a wimp." John suggested to me that my attempts to "rise above the fray" were really sinking points for my emotional well-being. "That may be so," I countered, "but Phil's mood swings and grandiosity were mental health problems that I didn't understand—and neither did Phil, for that matter." John seemed to accept my testimony. He laughed when I recalled thinking long ago that Phil was a turkey with no feathers, a lot of strut and naked vulnerability.

Over dinner John apologized for "coming after me." He was honest that he thought Jena's and my Christian beliefs were an empty well. I made no apology for believing in a loving God who informed the way I tried to live. Perhaps John was consciously or even unconsciously testing my willingness to fight. I got the clear idea from him that my willingness to battle was critical to my well-being. I didn't think I was a pushover then or ever really had been. It was true I didn't seek adversaries, and in an adversarial circumstance I always tried to ask myself, "What's going on?" before I started swinging.

Alzheimer's was an inescapable adversary, patiently waiting for my return to Minnesota. Phil's new difficulty in remembering how to sit down gave me an idea for his Christmas gift. His old swivel chair had become a problem. He'd missed the seat several times when it had spun to the side. Staff had called me to report his falls. Recently I'd found him crossways on his bed, where I assumed he'd sat instead. His body had tipped over backwards, and his head rested at right angles against the wall. He looked miserably uncomfortable.

I went to the La-Z-Boy store and sat in dozens of recliners. Phil and I were about the same height at that point. He seemed to be shrinking before my eyes. I figured what was comfortable to my frame would serve him well. Long rows of options filled the barnlike store. I chose a supple leather chair that did not swivel but pushed back easily. My body fit the soft, well-padded arms and headrest in a kind of nest.

The new chair was a hit. Not so the 2007 Wellstead Christmas party. The live country and western singers were too loud for Phil. He told me, "Turn them off!" Back in his room he sat in his new chair and accepted shoulder rubs with Andrea Bocelli singing holiday songs softly on public radio. Our own intimate Christmas party soothed both of us.

Leaving Wellstead, I had conditioned myself to set Phil aside and reenter life in our broader family. Everyone was in town, including Mother. When the packages were passed from the tree, there was a present to me from Phil. "He would want to give you a present," Mother explained. Her thoughtful gesture was meant well. It definitely broke through my reserve. I choked out, "Thank you." Phil hadn't understood wrapped gifts for a long time, either the receiving or the giving of them. Our connection with his new chair had been gift enough.

That Phil never left Wellstead during the holidays was sadder for us than for him. We all went to see him in small groups. He was so pleased with the cherry pie that Jena brought to him that he fed it to himself, a skill which by that time he had mostly lost.

The night before Jena's family departed, she and I found ourselves alone in my laundry room. For the first time, she asked me, "Mom, what would you do?" Part of me had longed for that moment, that opportunity, that responsibility to give advice on marital troubles. Nonetheless, I heard myself saying, "I think I know what I might do, but I am not you. Only you can decide what you will do." I assured her once again of my love and went off to bed thinking, "Damn. Wasn't there something more helpful I could have said?" As I ruminated and wept, I was drawn back to Pastor Van Dyke's Christmas Eve sermon. He said that the importance of receiving is manifested in the birth of Christ, a wondrous gift for humankind. How to notice it, to accept it, to sing its praise, to live a life informed by it was, is, and always will be a worthy challenge in the presence of busy lives. Phil was hardly the Christ child, but I saw him as a gift. I wondered if Jena might see her Marc as a gift.

In the flurry of her early morning departure, I found a moment to give her this image: "Think of Marc as a gift, not necessarily what you had expected or hoped for but special all the same." I immediately worried that the image was not helpful in her case. We hugged good-bye.

I entered the new year of 2008 living my solo country life and tending the remnants of Phil's and my relationship. I gave up trying to figure things out and took up Viktor Frankl's counsel. In *Man's Search for Meaning* he says, "We need to stop asking about the meaning of life, and instead to think of ourselves as those who are being questioned by life—daily and hourly." Making sense with my head in the clouds and my heart in my throat was not enough. Life required a "knees in the dirt" response.

At Wellstead, two of the residents in Phil's unit had recently died. Two others had moved to a different unit because their capacities had become so diminished. Phil no longer paid much attention to the others anyway. The previous year's lunch conversations had disappeared. For me, the storytelling had allowed fond recollection. I had sung Phil's praises as a skilled hunter and game cooker, conjuring up the scene at Phil's duck hunting club in Hugo. I had described hundreds of ducks circling the marsh and our hunting dog shivering with excitement waiting for Phil's occasional gunshot. Phil would take perfect aim. Splash! Then he would holler, "Dead bird," sending the dog crashing into the icy water to retrieve it. Some of the guys had joined in with their own stories.

Now Phil and I left a silent table and retired to his quiet room. I pushed the play button for us to enjoy Michael Feinstein CDs. The romantic tunes brought a warm memory of a different kind to me. Staff would close Phil's door so none of the ambulatory residents would bother us. It was a simple time together: nothing planned, expected, or hoped for. I even dozed sometimes.

One day I stopped at Maynard's and brought lunch to Phil. I was hungry. The restaurant boxed up halibut fingers, tartar sauce, filet mignon, and fresh fruit. I was not sure what might appeal to him. His appetite was disappearing. The food smelled good, though, and he did not turn his head away as I offered small bites.

I had a hard time knowing what to talk about with him. I couldn't mention our grandson Tom's recent hockey game. Phil no longer went with me to those games. The cold winter wind scared him. One step out the door, he would close his eyes and pull his head into his jacket collar like a turtle into its shell. I still loved the games. In the Saint Mary's Point/Hudson contest, Tom had scored the winning goal.

Afterwards his dad, the coach, encouraged me to go into the locker room and congratulate him. At age ten, Tom was unembarrassed by family fans. Red faced and sweating, he was sitting on a bench undoing his skates. Seeing me, he jumped up with a smile and allowed a big hug. I was so proud of him and the whole team. After the game, stopping the car at the first traffic light, I burst into tears. I had to pull over and collect myself from a riptide of emotion where Alzheimer's lurked.

I'd long ago given up attempting church with Phil as well. The next morning I went by myself. It was announced that the associate pastor would be in the small Elizabeth Chapel between services to pray with any member who might like such special time. Darlene was my friend, the one who had married Heidi and baptized the grandchildren. Other parishioners went to coffee hour, or enrichment, or home. My feet took me to the Elizabeth Chapel that morning. Only Darlene was there when I came in. I went forward. She asked me, "Oh, Barbara, how are you? How is Phil?" I said softly, "We're okay," but tears streamed down my face. In flood I told her that this week marked the fourth anniversary of Dad's death, that Jena and Marc were likely divorcing, that their kids did not know yet, that Phil's weight was dropping, that I'd burst into unexpected tears at the traffic light, that needing help for myself was painful, and on and on.

I had supposed that Saturday's tears were for Phil because he could no longer attend the children's games. Suddenly I admitted that they were for me. Watching the hockey kids give their all, I'd witnessed one of my highest values in action: try hard! "Trying hard doesn't matter," I lamented. "Alzheimer's is long and arduous, not just for the afflicted. No matter what I do, Alzheimer's advances, and poor Phil declines. I'm exhausted." Darlene hugged me and said a beautiful prayer, asking God's help for me. When I turned to go, others had seated themselves in the pews. I'd been standing before them in public confession. I smiled weakly and left feeling lighter.

During the next week I stayed home some days, taking it easy. Pitching old files and reading cleared the air somewhat. I didn't always add a visit to Wellstead when I went into town for a meeting. When I was pinched for time one day after lunch with Abby and friends, she asked me, "Are you going as a duty?" I discounted her implication, responding, "I like to spend time with Phil." I did. I also no longer tried to stuff quite so much into my schedule. Leaving Abby, as I reached the highway, I could go west to Rogers or east to St. Mary's Point. I went home.

The next day I went to see Phil. He recognized me immediately. I brought him juicy seedless grapes and Mariah. She jumped onto his lap. He caressed her fur. Out of the blue, he said, "I love you." We walked loops inside his unit, holding hands. The aide watched us. "Barbara, he's so happy when you're here," she exclaimed. The nurse chimed in, "He's been a bit vacant the last few days." I chose to hear that my presence could elevate Phil's experience and not to dwell on his blankness at other times. I too had experienced the blankness of being lost to him. I no longer expected his delight, but I surely enjoyed it.

Beyond Wellstead, February 2008 was a sad time. Jena's children, Max and Mimi, were much in my heart. Ages thirteen and twelve, they would soon learn that Mom and Dad were ending their marriage. What remained for the adults was to go forward as loving parents. That was their promise. What remained for the children was less clear. I prayed that they would know that they were truly loved and would be able to trust love. I agonized at their having to cope with the loss of their parents' marriage. I was mature and could scarcely bear my own loss of Phil to Alzheimer's.

What if Phil and I had divorced years earlier? I was glad that we had not. Whether because of Phil and me or in spite of us, our children had all grown into wonderful adults. They were the greatest gifts of Phil's and my marriage. Certainly Jena and Marc felt the same way about Max and Mimi. I trusted that these precious children would be all right, wanting to offer them any part that I could play in helping to make that true.

I wrote Max and Mimi a letter, a copy for each in separate envelopes. I phoned each individually as well. Max acknowledged receiving my letter. His response was brief, but I felt he'd heard me. Sitting in the car in the Wellstead parking lot, I finally tracked down Mimi on my cell phone. In that place in that moment I told her that I didn't know why life was so hard. I wished her grandpa hadn't gotten sick. "Most days I do fine," I told her. "Then sometimes, at odd or surprising moments the sadness springs out at me, and I weep. Maybe that's how it will be for you." She told me a bit about her two new rooms, one at Mom's and one at Dad's. I told her I hoped she'd always feel at home wherever she was. She said her friends were being great to her. "Trust your feelings and tell your parents, too," I urged.

My good friend Sandy Kiernat invited me out for supper. She bravely asked me, "What will you do when Phil is no longer here?" That would be the final loss. I didn't know the answer. Keep being me, I supposed. That's what I hoped for my grandchildren, too, that they would continue to grow into themselves—with hope, with passion, and with compassion.

Spring came. Two fat doves stood on the stucco ledge outside my office window. They cooed and bobbed their heads at each other, reminding me we were entering the season of pairs. Out at Wellstead, Phil's cooing and bobbing were rarities. Chris came home. Together we went to see his dad. Phil was flat. No promising shoots of recognition or pleasure poked through the wintry crust of his Alzheimer's. I asked the aide how Phil had been that morning. She reported that he was in fine spirits and confided, "He initiated holding my arm, kissed me on the cheek, and said he loved me." Jesse was a bubbly young woman studying to become a nurse. Most of me was glad that Phil could appreciate what a great gal she was. I was also aware that I was growing less essential to him. I understood this circumstance was just another unhappy page in the book of Alzheimer's stories.

Chris and I stayed, but the visit had no real beginning, middle, or end for Phil. He did not greet us or really acknowledge being with us or bid us farewell. Like the frozen, colorless river, the scene offered no prospect of spring. We left disappointed. "Mom, how do you keep going?" Chris asked, sighing. "Some days are better than others," I replied. "Not a lot better, but certainly better," I thought to myself. Life on the tundra was spare.

# CHAPTER 14

Accepting Change

Nearly twenty months into Phil's stay at Wellstead, I was torn between thinking that I no longer had special value to him and that I needed to summon more imagination and courage to find new ways of relating to him. The truth was that I simply showed up for my two-hour visits and experienced whatever happened. Sometimes I even glanced at my watch to see if my two hours were up. I could not be spontaneous in visiting, as the long drive to Wellstead required timing. In the spring of 2008 the road crews were hard at work repairing the interstate, which made avoiding rush hour all the more critical.

One day I pushed toward Rogers after the Wilder Foundation's Audit Committee meeting and another organization's fundraising luncheon. I'd not been thinking about Phil except that Wellstead was the third activity on my day's agenda. Phil was crumpled on his bed sideways, his new chair vacant. I put on soft music and took his hand in mine. Snuggling up to him, I smelled his Old Spice deodorant. I didn't study his face for understanding. Rather like one of our pups, I simply went to him.

My poor sweetheart could not get up by himself. Together we eventually got him to a standing position. He stared blankly at his room, as if to see where he was, and wandered into the common area. I gently stepped beside him and took his hand again. That pressure returned his attention to me. We walked to the pond across the street and watched the red-winged blackbirds flitting among the cattails. Pointing to a swimming duck, I could not direct Phil's attention to it. He was no longer able to switch focus at will. Our pleasure in wildlife had lost its mutuality. Still, the fresh air felt good. And in my hands, I considered Phil safe.

I was never sure what he was thinking or if he could think in any traditional way. His language, mostly single words by this time, often seemed unrelated to the experience at hand. Hearing him say, "River," I was shocked. He had not been out to the St. Croix River for ten months, and he had long before stopped begging to go home. I agonized, remembering the picnics on Heidi's deck the previous summer. The slim possibility that he longed to be with me in our house haunted me anew. I had taken odd comfort in the notion that Phil did not know what he was missing. I counted on his lack of memory as a protection against wretched feelings of disappointment.

When Beth visited before Memorial Day, she was resigned to the idea that her dad no longer remembered her. Entering Phil's unit, we were pleased to find a musician playing guitar and singing. Her little girls immediately entered the circle of residents and danced to the music. Everyone was amused. With Phil smiling broadly, I imagined grandfatherly pleasure, which was a stretch. I couldn't help wishing for him to enjoy pride in his progeny.

Weather permitting, Heidi and I wanted to bring Phil home on Father's Day. Our plan was for me to stay home and make a light lunch while she drove the two-hour round trip to Rogers to collect Phil. Rob would bring the children over to see us at my house, but they would not stay for lunch. I would keep the dogs confined in their kennel, walk Phil to the river, serve him lunch, and drive back.

The day dawned brilliantly, and the plan went into action. Excited by Phil's homecoming, I chopped fruit and prepared deviled eggs in a happy dance around my kitchen. Heidi predicted that Phil would not know where he was, but anticipating him in his own setting meant a lot to me. My bridegroom was coming!

When Heidi drove into the driveway, I ran to the car to open his door. With assistance, he was soon standing on his own land. We didn't go inside, but rather set off on a slow walk down the grassy path toward

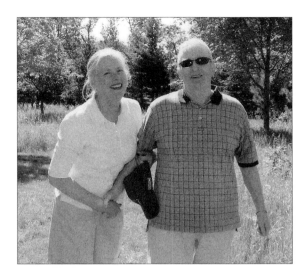

*Phil and me on Father's Day, 2008*

the river. Holding onto my arm, Phil managed the bumpy terrain and seemed to take pleasure in whatever fell into his sight line: early wild-flowers, birds on wing, shady nooks. I spoke with enthusiasm about the river but could not steer him close enough to it that he ever took its notice. Rob and the children appeared, grandson Tom took photos of Phil and me walking hand in hand, and we all settled on the deck. Phil fell immediately to sleep. Heidi cushioned the metal chair arms and wrapped a blanket around his shoulders. Then she placed her sunglasses on Phil's face. The children surrounded him for one last photo and left quietly.

Heidi and I looked at each other. Phil was too tired to eat. I packed our lunch to take it back to Wellstead. We gently roused her dad and got him into my car so he could nap on the drive back. He did not say good-bye. Heidi bid me a heartfelt farewell, and off I drove.

Back at Wellstead, while I was setting up our lunch at the kitchen counter, out of the corner of my eye I saw Phil wander into another man's bathroom. In a split second he fell. I ran and lay down beside him. The nurse came to assess the situation. Fortunately Phil was unperturbed and uninjured. We soon sat down together at the kitchen counter for our picnic. Phil ate eagerly, including the cherry pie that staff had saved for him. For a time we watched golf on TV. When I announced I had to go feed Sunny, Phil smooched and released me.

He had no idea of others' feelings and effort that had gone into his trip home. But, somehow, I sensed that he had had a fine day. A sunny walk was great while he was walking. Rides were pleasant in the comfort of Heidi's and my cars. The food piqued his appetite. His fall was forgotten almost immediately. All was well for him. I was recomforted by the notion that he did not know what he was missing at the river and that he was where he belonged. What if he had fallen in our meadow?

The following Wednesday, a funeral director was pushing a gurney out of Phil's unit when I arrived. His neighbor Carl had died, the sixth man since January. Carl's loving family members were frequent visitors like us. We often chatted with each other and with each other's loved one in residence. I offered my condolences and recounted a recent visit that included our son, when scrawny Carl had sat with us. I had told Chris, "Carl has a fine family." Carl had smiled and responded, "They better be!" Glad for the story, his daughter Kathy mused, "That's vintage Dad speaking!"

Phil did not take direct note of the death of others, seemingly indifferent to who was gone or who was new. Perhaps he no longer understood death as our shared fate. Still, he registered change in the atmosphere. He giggled, frowned, and muttered, "Fuck," as he circled the courtyard carrying a footstool. He didn't eat well. His odd behavior was sad on a sad day.

Phil's general withdrawal included disinterest in meals. In September 2008 his athletic, muscular body lost five pounds. I often brought him raspberries, for which he opened his mouth like a baby bird. However, staff often now wrote 50 percent or less on his meal consumption chart. The wasting effect of Alzheimer's was underway. Forgetting how to use utensils, difficulty with accepting being fed, and loss of appetite—all were contributing to Phil's weight loss.

His loss of robust appearance and strength coincided with a shift from his aggressive behavior to being the target of several newcomers. One fellow pushed him down. Another guy approached Phil, who was seated for supper, and grabbed his head from behind. Staff had to break up the hammerlock. Phil's wandering path frequently took him too close to Sterling, who enjoyed sticking his foot out. Phil went flying numerous times. He cut his forehead and jammed his glasses into his nose. Luckily, he didn't break any bones. By regulation, every infraction was reported to me. I hated thinking about Phil's vulnerability, and I hated receiving the phone calls that confirmed it.

On a rare night out with Abby, she naturally inquired how I was. "I don't hurt," I responded thinking of Phil's crashes. My second summer of family visitors was winding down. How I was seemed secondary to my concentration on the rest of my tribe. That Phil was ill, that Mother was old, and that three of my children lived away were facts that framed much of what was important to me. I cherished the time I had with them. "I'm not getting the exercise I need," I admitted. "I'm not exactly an old tub bobbing in the waves, nor am I a sleek sailboat in full sail. I'm more of a kayak, not suited for big water, but agile enough in shallow streams close to the life that grows there." She eyed me with loving suspicion.

By the end of September, it was Phil's turn to move to a different unit within Wellstead for his protection and in recognition of his further deterioration. He was beginning to fall without provocation. I dreaded the move as a symbol more than as an event. The new unit was definitely home to the trees in winter that Anne Lamott alluded to. Very few of the residents were ambulatory. Several of them groaned and screamed in the winds of disease. Most of the new faces were expressionless. One fellow regularly regurgitated his meal onto his bib, which didn't fully protect his clothes or the table where he sat. Many meals were pureed beyond distinction to prevent choking. There was no interaction between residents.

The only good news was that Bob Simpson lived there, and Anne visited him frequently. Sometimes Bob and Phil were assigned to the same table. Anne and I could chat with each other as we fed our husbands, which gave our table a bit of cordiality. Blind, Bob could still recognize Anne's voice. Still somewhat social, Phil could absorb pleasant conversational tones. We treated our men with tender dignity and utmost respect. We didn't complain, roll our eyes, or throw up our hands as one spouse did. I put a smile on my face, a lilt in my voice, and a bounce in my step when I saw Phil. As surprising as it was to most others not in our situation, Anne and I took pleasure in the possibility of connecting with Bob and Phil. Connecting was still a real if unpredictable gift.

The staff in the new unit remained friendly and caring. Phil had no adjustment to make in that regard. His room was configured slightly differently. His chair now sat by the window and looked back toward his door that opened onto the common area. He could watch the sparse activity in the unit, and staff could easily see him sitting in his room.

I was glad for improved safety until one day when, once I arrived, no one could find him. He wasn't in his room. He wasn't in the common area. He'd not escaped into the sunroom, following another family through the temporarily unlocked door. He hadn't fallen behind a couch. Where was he? Why hadn't anyone noticed his absence?

Phil had inadvertently closed himself into the bathroom. When I opened the door, he was facing the back wall as if it were a dead end. He had not known how to turn around or get out. I'd been searching for him for what seemed a long time. I didn't know how long he'd been there before I began my search. He was not agitated, but I was. He might have been left there until lunch and collapsed in exhaustion. "You need to know where Phil is at all times," I reprimanded the staff gently. "He deserves to be cared for, not just brought out for meals!" The incident taught staff about both Phil and me. Even though his gait was stiff, Phil still liked to move around. He needed watching. And even though my concern was well founded, I was not blaming. I relied on and appreciated the people who worked at Wellstead.

Then two days later, my phone rang at three a.m. Phil had had a seizure. His screams had drawn the nursing assistant to his room. His body was jumping spasmodically in his bed with his eyes rolling. He'd been unresponsive to her voice or touch. So she'd immediately called the night nurse, who quickly came to see Phil and contacted his internist for appropriate medication. Phil had come out of the seizure naturally, but he was exhausted. At last, the nurse called me with her report, saying, "Phil will likely sleep for hours. Don't hurry to come."

I could not return to sleep. I showered, forced myself to eat breakfast, packed a bag, emailed Heidi to call me on my cell phone when she awakened, and set off in the dark for Rogers. Tiny in the black landscape peppered by oncoming truck headlights, I wondered, "Is this how it ends? Phil alone and me helplessly trying to reach him?"

When I finally shut the motor off in the dark parking lot, my shoulders slumped against the steering wheel. I felt like a discarded sandbag useless against the ravages of flood.

This perilous experience was far worse than the flood of 1997 on the St. Croix River. Then advanced warnings from the Army Corps of Engineers and the old high-water mark in the summerhouse closet told us what to expect. The summerhouse first floor would go under. The Hennesseys, who had bought the summerhouse from us, moved their furniture to the second floor and stayed in town, where they lived during most of the year.

Phil and I thought we were ready. When we built our new riverfront house, code required our main floor to be two feet above the 1965 high-water mark. We'd installed drains in the basement closets in case of flood. By the hour, day, and week, the water rose as predicted. We stayed put, moving everything out of the basement into the garage and the cars out to the road. We bought sump pumps.

In reality we were quickly overwhelmed. Our septic system was incapacitated before the water even got in the house. We didn't realize that the water would come up and stay. Receding more slowly than it had risen to its crest, it sat there and defied any expectation it would return to normal. For weeks, our house was nearly surrounded by water with only a camp stool in the garage for relief. I carried our waste out daily in what I called the family colostomy bag. Two feet of water stood in the basement. It had not come through windows or doors but through the cement floor.

Wearing my fishing waders, I patrolled the basement to monitor the sump pumps. They shot the rising water out the windows to buy time before more water would seep through the floor. Keeping the water depth at a certain level was important to prevent the cement from buckling. I was the captain of reverse pressure, and I had no manual for the tedious assignment.

Similarly, during Phil's two years at Wellstead I'd monitored Alzheimer's progression and fought against it with scaled-back, doable activities and tender care. Like the rising river, however, the disease was immutable. There was no stopping it or pushing it back. Unlike the river, its pressure and presence would never subside until death cut Phil free. Still, I did not want him to die. I wasn't ready to let him go.

I went inside. Much to my relief, Phil's eyes fluttered open when I kissed his forehead. Whether he knew me I did not know, but he'd responded. He cooperated with the nurse's efforts to collect new blood pressure and pulse readings, both of which had returned to normal. Then he dozed off again. I collapsed into his recliner.

Over the course of the next week, as the doctors ramped up Phil's antiseizure medication, he was wobbly, dopey, and less himself. Heidi, the doctors, and I conferred. Struggling to choose and balance Phil's medication was not a new challenge. With patient experimentation, we eventually got Phil on his feet again.

The next month I dared to join my daughters in Boston to celebrate Heidi's fortieth birthday. We all owed Heidi a debt of gratitude for her constancy in tending Phil, but more we wanted to salute her new decade and loving spirit. In all the heartache of Phil's decline, it remained important to me to continue to celebrate the goodness of life. Laughter and real companionship lightened my soul.

When I came home from Boston after just four days, seeing Phil was a shock. Curled up under a comforter on top of his single bed, he looked so small. I pulled up a chair and took his hand. We stayed like that for almost an hour trading quiet smiles. He gave no sign of wanting to get up. I wanted to curl up with him, but I was afraid I might scare him. I felt awkward and too big.

When I did try to help him up, he was as stiff as driftwood. He couldn't automatically relax his muscles, and my gentle efforts could not unbend him. Down another five pounds, his withered, fragile frame was frozen almost beyond recognition.

His eyes told me that he wanted to get up, so I persisted in trying to right him. Finally on his feet, he lurched forward as if propelled by an invisible windup mechanism. "Okay, Phil, let's slow down a bit," I offered, stepping in front of him to prevent his toppling over. He leaned heavily on me, and together we managed a dozen steps that led to his special chair. As usual I put on some soft music. Phil closed his eyes and relaxed his hand in mine, our fingers keeping time. After a while, I slipped away to dip some ice cream, which he willingly accepted in blind spoonfuls. Giving him such small pleasure gave me huge pleasure. Then came the miracle of his whole, coherent sentence: "I'm so glad when I can make you happy!"

The words sparkled in truth for both of us. It's hard to know for sure where they came from. God's loving spirit within Phil? I was stunned. I wished Phil could hold and savor that thought as I would. Maybe deep inside he did.

Weeks later, out of nowhere, he greeted me from the lunch table, "You're sexy." The staff and I laughed aloud to Phil's further delight. I sat down beside him, but he would not eat. On our customary walk around the unit, he began to sob. Anne intercepted us, tenderly asking Phil, "Are you scared?" Bob was often scared; he was blind and generally unable to do anything for himself. Maybe Phil was scared. He couldn't tell me. He didn't have the words. He'd never really had words to talk about being afraid.

Instead, like the time he'd run the *Argonauta* into the wing dam, I just held him in my arms and rocked him. Sitting side by side on a sunny sofa, I spoke softly to him about how much his family loved him. Forty-five minutes of my whispering and stroking his shoulders melted us into one another. I despaired leaving him after such an emotional exchange. His current anguish contrasted so starkly with his miraculous sentence of gladness expressed weeks earlier. I wanted to keep my reassuring hand on him. I prayed for a higher Constant Hand to hold Phil and for him to feel that presence.

In December Heidi's loving hand found Phil more diminished. "Mom, Dad's weight is down to 150 pounds. His face is puckered. He doesn't seem to be having a very good day," she reported from Wellstead. "It is what it is," she concluded. I could hear her talking to herself and needing to confide in me. We were both thinking more about Phil dying than we had in the past.

How long did he have to suffer? How many bad days did he have to endure? How much sadness could we all absorb? I did not know the answers. In spite of Phil's illness we were carrying on. The holidays and all the family were coming. We couldn't spend our time waiting for Phil to die. As far as I was concerned, we honored him by living our lives, having fun together as a family, and just holding his hand. His human flame still flickered. We knew not what would douse it or when. Heidi asked me, "Will you be sad or relieved when Dad dies?" I responded, "Both, I imagine."

My good friend Joanna's sister Linda had received her Alzheimer's diagnosis years before Phil had, and she was still hanging on. When Jo came to see Phil before Christmas, she brought her mother's Norwegian *kringler*. The almond fragrance and her kind face drew his attention. "How's that?" she asked slipping a small, sweet bite into his mouth. Phil nodded and opened his mouth for more. "Dear Philemon, we've had so much fun," she continued, gaily recounting old stories of our boating trips together as couples. He clearly felt her friendship. She thought she heard him say, "Arna," his pet name for her, and her eyes filled. He accepted our support for several leisurely loops of the unit before retiring in his recliner. He was worn out. He'd worked very hard to participate. I pushed the lever to elevate his feet, covered him with a blanket, and kissed him good-bye. His eyes were already closed.

Outside his room Jo waited for me with unquenched tears. My dear husband was so different from the Philemon in her stories. Visiting Phil five days a week, I had seen his changes in slow motion. Cumulatively they were not in his favor. Nevertheless, on a daily basis, bright moments like the one with Joanna broke through. Our children and Mother all visited Phil over the holidays with mixed results. Sometimes he was too sleepy to participate. Sometimes he sat slouched to one side like a poorly packed sack of potatoes. Sometimes his legs would give out unexpectedly. Other times he appeared to listen to conversation, and occasionally he interjected a word. Family members won Phil's smiles, laughter, and hand squeezes. I wove my own solo visits into the mix as well, no longer aspiring to being a fresh, bright light in his existence. I was his constant. To the extent he could count on me, I wanted him to do so.

# CHAPTER 15

## Enriching My Life

Phil soldiered on hour by hour and day by day, and I continued to enter into his world faithfully. The year 2009 began with the inauguration of President Barack Obama. I turned on the television for Phil and me to watch the proceedings together. Politics aside, Obama was a fine orator. He concluded his speech this way:

> So let us mark this day with remembrance, of who we are and how far we have traveled. In the year of America's birth, in the coldest months, a small band of patriots huddled by dying campfires on the shores of an icy river. The capital was abandoned. The enemy was advancing. The snow was stained with blood. At a moment when the outcome of our revolution was most in doubt, the father of our nation ordered these words be read to the people: "Let it be told to the future world . . . that in the depth of winter, when nothing but hope and virtue could survive . . . that the city and the country, alarmed at one common danger, came forth to meet [it]."
>
> America, in the face of our common dangers, in this winter of our hardship, let us remember these timeless words. With hope and virtue, let us brave once more the icy currents and endure what storms may come. Let it be said by our children's children that when we were tested we refused to let this journey end, that we did not turn back nor did we falter; and with eyes fixed on the horizon

and God's grace upon us, we carried forth that great gift of freedom and delivered it safely to future generations.

I was aroused by the message and turned to Phil. He looked at me, and although he had not spoken a full sentence in months, he asked, "What can I do?" Whether his emotive self had taken some meaning from the speech, I didn't know. Perhaps he was just asking what we were going to do next. I hugged him and said, "Stick with me, baby." My spontaneous words were definitely an emotional response to Phil's presence, to the president's words, and to my deep belief in working through the challenges that life presented.

That evening I ate my supper alone with the TV continuing inaugural coverage. When the camera turned to the inaugural balls and fell on the First Couple dancing, I wept. Phil and I were good dancers. I missed our effortless steps and warm embraces, the shared beat and the fun.

In late January, I joined old Minnesota friends in Florida to play golf and relax. I eagerly accepted the opportunity for friendship and warm sunshine. The day before I left, I visited Phil and received an unexpected gift: another full sentence. Looking into my eyes, he whispered, "We're not over yet." It was a sweet affirmation. Phil did not know about my planned trip, and his words did not hold me back.

Returning after six days, my longest break from Phil at Wellstead, I did feel guilty. Had I been unfaithful to my pledge to be Phil's constant? I took his lack of attention to me as purposeful aloofness. Attributing his behavior to my absence was rather silly, but I couldn't help it. Most likely he simply didn't remember me right away. On my second visit, Phil was comfortable with me again. Eating the cold blueberries and sliced apples I brought, we reconnected. Staff assisted me in getting him out of his chair. We walked into the sunroom arm in arm, and he nodded kindly to others. Seeing him brighten and interact warmly with others gave me a sense that he was all right. I left him in the care of two aides, who were gently guiding him into his bathroom before lunch.

The next Sunday Phil developed focal motor seizures. Sitting next to him, mindlessly watching television, I felt his hand start to jerk. His whole right side became spastic, contorting and flailing about uncontrollably. As thankful as I was to be with him in the moment, I didn't know what to do. Staff had never seen anything like it. When the Wellstead nurse finally came, she called Phil's doctor. Waiting for new medication to arrive, I was glad Phil could not see himself. His appearance and condition were terrifying. Continuing to hold his hand, I allowed mine to assume the crazy arm dance with him for three hours. I could only hope he was not in pain; he wasn't screaming out. His eyes were wide and vacant. My feeling of powerlessness totally sapped me.

On Monday the focal motor seizures returned. Dr. Holm called with three options: do nothing, do blood work and adjust the current anti-seizure medication, or institute Ativan as needed to stop the seizures. He told me that the seizures themselves were not life threatening. I opted for Ativan. I wanted the seizures stopped as quickly as possible.

Tuesday there were more but milder seizures. Staff needed clarification on how often to give the Ativan. I was under the impression that Ativan was an emergency order, not a casual "we don't want these jerks to escalate" order. By late afternoon, Dr. Holm finally spoke to the Wellstead nurse to specify the plan, and I dragged myself home.

I returned on Wednesday, my fifth consecutive visit. Phil experienced no seizures. I was relieved for his and my own sake. "How," I wondered, "did I go to see Phil six out of seven days his first year at Wellstead?" The strain of travel and constant witness to his new condition were grueling. When Phil fell asleep for his first nap in three days, I left. I met Anne Simpson for supper and a lecture on Islam at my church, House of Hope Presbyterian. I needed to switch gears. Once home I slept hard and determined not to go to Wellstead in the morning.

Instead I spent Thursday morning on my computer tending the details of Phil's potential move to Boutwells Landing in Stillwater. This senior community was only twelve miles from my house. Presbyterian Homes was just finishing a new wing that included a nursing home for folks suffering from dementia. Having Phil closer to home with medical care on site was very appealing. He was definitely no longer a threat to fellow residents. The opening date was uncertain, however, and others already living in the Boutwells Landing community had priority. I wanted Phil's name as high as possible on the new admissions list.

I was the triage person, connecting Phil's doctors, Wellstead staff, and my caregiving observations to the new facility. But I had trouble achieving professional efficiency. I was easily distracted, scrambling for contact information, running to the bathroom, shepherding the dogs in and out, and accepting multiple calls from a cherished friend in Chicago who was in high excitement about planning a get-together. I almost forgot to make my own lunch before heading to an afternoon strategic planning meeting at the Wilder Foundation.

On Friday I returned to Wellstead. Phil seemed in no distress. He enjoyed the raspberries I brought. Could I dare to think we were back in a routine? That night I made myself a nice dinner and plopped on my couch to watch a movie before bed. Before turning out the light I made the mistake of trying a few games of Solitaire on my computer. The very name of the game lowered my spirits. I lost and refused to quit until I won. When I won, I wanted to win again. It was so hard for me to relax.

Over the next several months I broke away twice for long weekends, one in Florida for a golf tournament and one in San Francisco to hang out with Beth's family. My special Florida friend had been improving her golf game over the five years I'd been gone. She shot an 88. My golf was lousy, but it only mattered on the scorecard. On the West Coast my grandbabies were terrific. Cait was already five, and Imogen four. It seemed so long ago when they were born in New York City. Their personalities were blossoming. I tried not to think of their vibrant development in contrast to Phil's decline. We girls hiked in the Muir Woods, galloped through the Discovery Museum, and danced in Miss Kitty's music program. Magically transported, I thoroughly enjoyed myself and let go of Phil's needs.

In late March Phil gave me another of his word gifts. On a particularly alert day for him, we strolled into the sunroom and found a gentleman playing the piano for his mom. Phil had lost the agility that he displayed in our earlier Wellstead dance, but he still had rhythm. The toe-tapping tunes put some bounce in our step as we paced the length of the room over and over again.

When we settled back in his room, I said, "You are Dr. Roy." He said, "Right." Smiling at him, I continued, "And I am Mrs. Roy." He kept looking at me and responded, "That's perfect!" My smile grew bigger. He raised his hand and placed it on my head. That he wanted to reach out to me and actually did was a thrill.

Wellstead staff appreciated Phil's and my strong relationship and understood that we needed to leave their care. With Heidi's ever-present help we made the move to Boutwells Landing at the end of April 2009. Sitting at the kitchen counter with other residents, Phil noticed neither our packing up his room nor the movers hauling his belongings out of the unit to their waiting truck. "Phil, we're going on a trip," I then told him. Wellstead staff helped get his Golden Gophers jacket on him, walked with us to Heidi's car, sat him in the back seat, and swung his legs into a forward facing position. Heidi pushed the power door shut and headed her car out of the entrance we'd first come in that fateful day in August 2006. Phil sat peacefully next to me, looking out the window onto the gray, sunless landscape.

When we pulled up to the new facility in Stillwater forty-five minutes later, three smiling helpers greeted us cordially. Phil responded to their friendly presence, indifferent to the movers ahead of us carrying his things inside. He walked trustingly into the building, into the elevator, and into the third-floor memory care unit. He sat down in his own chair in his new room and watched as Heidi and I put away his belongings. Heidi went on her way, and I stayed for lunch.

The table was set with linens and stemware. We were the only guests in the dining room. We were meant to feel special, and I did. Phil sat straight in his chair and had a good appetite for a change. When we returned to his room, I completed paperwork with staff. Phil held a piece of paper too, still awake to the conversation about him. Official tasks done, I turned on the CD player, and Phil fell asleep. I was tired too, grateful that I faced only the twelve-mile ride home.

I'd caught a sudden cold. My head was leaden. I put myself to bed for a two-hour nap. The move couldn't have been easier in the end, but we'd been working toward it for several weeks.

Little steps like throwing out torn clothing, discarding the children's artwork, simplifying Phil's photo collection, reviewing his toiletries—I had done all of that while he snoozed during my visits. Buying fresh T-shirts, new khakis, missing toiletries, and room supplies—I had filled the shopping cart at Target with everything I could think of. Heidi's daughters, ages nine and eight, had decorated the new room with welcoming and loving pictures. We all wanted Grandpa to have a happy, fresh start.

Phil's adjustment was trouble free. The atmosphere, if not familiar, was immediately positive. One of the first residents to move in, Phil benefitted from extra staff time. They thought he was a sweetheart, and he was. He cooperated with their care and liked the tasty food. Staff could not have imagined Phil's requiring six helpers to get him into his first shower at Wellstead.

I benefitted from his proximity. If I found him deeply asleep on the first try of a given day, I'd come back. I skipped some days, suffering less angst because I knew that I could be there in fifteen minutes if staff called. Some days I visited at suppertime, using a whole day for my own enterprises and allowing our day's end to conclude in companionship. I enjoyed working in the yard again. I dug into the strategic planning effort underway at the Wilder Foundation. Not fighting construction and freeway traffic two and half hours per trip was a huge gift of time.

In June I made a bold move: I went to Japan. It was Beth's idea. Being invited to join her family on a big adventure was both heart warming and mind stretching. How could I fly eleven hours away from Phil? Heidi encouraged me to go for it. With her dad close by, she promised to multiply her visits. She reminded me, "There have been no more seizures. Dad's mood is good. The new team at Boutwells Landing is very attentive."

I particularly enjoyed Kyoto. At the Zen Buddhist Ryōan-ji Temple, I bought myself a small remembrance. It was four interlocking characters that, according to our guide, formed the sentence, "I know enough." The characters represented the quieting of the mind, freeing it from distractions and external demands and thereby opening it to happiness. The message was a powerful reminder to me to claim the time to turn inward and find peace in such quiet.

The adjacent garden featured fifteen rocks placed in a rectangle of fine gravel. From no perspective on the perimeter could all fifteen rocks be seen at once. The garden was intended to invite imagination beyond what is seen. A wall separated this hardscape from the verdant garden where alternating rows of cherry and maple trees could display the changing seasons. The intentional contrast between permanence and change and between the visible and the unseen supposedly represented the complexity of life. The ancient site was a masterpiece of Japanese culture. I found it beautiful.

The trip was precious as family time too. While I was helpful in small ways on the trip, Beth took the lead in all planning. I followed along like a puddle duck, and that felt good. Together we three generations explored the grounds of the Silver Pavilion. As Cait and Imogen scampered along the paths, I wondered at a six-hundred-year-old tree that had survived with the pavilion. Time defied ordinary measure. I savored the tiny moment given to me. I was so fortunate to be in the bosom of my family, learning something new and experiencing beauty.

Phil was unchanged and somewhat indifferent to me on my return. Dear Heidi had visited him five times in my eight-day absence. The frequency was made slightly more convenient by the fact that she had to deliver her daughters to art class in Stillwater that week. Heidi's energy and deep affection for her dad must have felt good to him. She reported only one misstep. Walking the common area with her singing, "You are my sunshine," Phil had come to an unexpected halt. His pants had fallen down. She hoisted them up, and they continued on their way.

On June 27 Beth called to check up on the Minnesota front. "It's Dad's and my forty-fifth wedding anniversary," I told her. "How old will you be when you and Oliver celebrate forty-five years?" She retorted, "I'm working on getting to ten years." In a fine mood myself, I replied, "Working on marriage is a great idea. Just remember to embrace each season." Perhaps I was talking to myself. Later at Boutwells Landing, Phil and I celebrated our anniversary listening to Tony Bennett sing "Smile." We could both still smile, "even though our hearts were breaking."

Jena, Max, and Mimi made their annual Fourth of July trip to Minnesota. Mother was in residence for the third summer. With Phil close by and an extra bedroom converted from his workshop, my houseful of family hummed. I kept loose track of a general plan of action. At ninety-seven, Mother delighted in the hubbub. As usual, Heidi hosted many picnics. Varying family teams provided Phil frequent visitors.

As Jena was leaving, Beth's team arrived. The little girls were delighted to go see Grandpa because he had a playground by his building. We loaded Phil into a wheelchair to ride on the walking path to the playground. There he sat to watch the girls climbing on the equipment. On one occasion he even managed to offer, "She's cute!"

Before Labor Day both Jena and Chris were in town. An outdoorsman himself, Chris liked seeing how the new place suited Phil's spirit. The morning light streamed into Phil's room, native plants adorned the courtyard, and lots of birds and butterflies flew about the walking path. Inside, he and Jena took turns on the small folding chair that I kept by Phil's recliner. I had learned that he had his best chance of connecting if I sat very close and at eye level. Watching them patiently win Phil's attention with soft words, I felt their loss and their love. Setting aside ordinary demands and concerns, they slipped tenderly into their dad's quiet space.

In October Phil's sister Allie made the trip from Dallas. Her big brother no longer looked very big. He was maintaining his weight, but he weighed less than 150 pounds. Asleep when we arrived, Phil swam languidly to the surface and eventually locked onto Allie sitting in the small folding chair. He looked at her intently as if trying to think who she might be. She took his hand, which gripped hers automatically as hard as a vise. Phil had lost his motor memory for unclenching. I rarely brought one of our dogs anymore because his squeezes made them yip with pain. Allie loved his surprise strength and grinned at him. I snapped a wonderful photo of them clutched together. Allie was gratified to find Phil reachable and at ease in their sweet time together.

Long ago the pressures of Phil's surgical career had often separated him from me and other family members. Many times I grew tired of Phil burying himself in business, whether medicine or yard work or sports or whatever he was doing. He had three speeds: intense work, brief silliness, and sleep. Now his doing was scant, but his eyes somehow invited a deeper connection, which we all treasured.

Allie and Phil had lost their mother in 1975. Allie liked having my mom dote on her during her stay with me. Mother was glad to extend her mothering, which included her worry, "You are not smoking, are you?!" Allie appreciated Mother's loving concern, too. The three of us bonded in a shopping expedition to buy fresh Tommy Bahama sweatshirts. My Texans were cold. They soon flew away.

On my own, after months of family in my house, I attended a wonderful Writing and Faith Conference at my church. The poet Scott Cairns told us that he wrote as a means to "apprehend what I do not know." I was stunned by the idea that he welcomed his own apprehensiveness and used poetry as a method of searching. Unlike the Ryōan-ji Temple characters that stilled the mind, he allowed his anxiety to open his mind. In both cases, though, turning inward was important. It wasn't selfish; it was soulful. I was ready for my own soulful time.

The headliner of the conference was Anne Lamott, the "trees in winter" author I admired. In our big sanctuary with towering stained-glass windows, she looked fragile, disorderly, and even out of place. A CD of her church's music blasted from the House of Hope sound system with a body pumping rhythm before she appeared looking like a newly hatched chick in a foreign barn. As she began to speak, she rambled. I remained hopeful that she'd find her footing, but felt a mild disappointment that she was "off." After a few minutes, she gained traction and told us that faith and writing are much the same, that they are about walking away from self-doubt.

I jotted down some of her "rules" and insights:

- Start where you are.
- Wing it.
- Courage is fear that's said its prayers.
- Slow down; multitasking is killing people.
- Be angry.
- Don't be afraid of mistakes. Fall into the abyss.
- Cry. It baptizes you.
- Meditate. Be quiet. This is where new instructions come.
- Learn to waste more time.

- Notice what's going on.
- Take a nap.
- Show up. Be willing to be miserable. God is there.

Without a note or an outline, she emptied her ragged sack of warm, loving advice with an easy generosity. I was touched. Her words were a brilliant code for the Alzheimer's journey.

In the long years of Phil's chronic illness, I had suffered with him. Falling deeper into the Alzheimer's abyss, I was no longer afraid that my mistakes mattered. I was learning to live better without any power to "put things right." Sharing tears and laughter was what mattered for all of us.

# CHAPTER 16

△▱▱▱△

# Looking Back

In early 2009, before we had moved Phil to Boutwells Landing, I received a long-distance call from the captain of Dartmouth's 1960 All Ivy Championship Hockey Team. He was inviting Phil and me to the team's upcoming fiftieth reunion. "I'm sorry. Phil and I cannot attend," I responded as usual. Rusty Ingersoll's enthusiasm quietly turned to compassionate concern when I told him that Phil was suffering from Alzheimer's. The celebratory idea of collecting the team members to enjoy their memories and catch up on the intervening years contrasted sharply with the reality of Phil's loss of memory and inability to tell his story. In the course of our warm phone conversation, I agreed to write a bio of Phil for the team's memory book, and Rusty invited me to Hanover on my own.

Certainly I knew Phil's athleticism, his delight in the game of hockey, and his pride in being a Dartmouth alum. The photograph he gave me to remember him, when I returned to Skidmore College in 1962, was of him in full Dartmouth hockey regalia. The eight-by-ten, black-and-white, official school photo portrayed Phil's preppie good looks in a confident pose. He had shoveled rinks on the river in front of our house so our children could skate. He had extricated himself from surgical responsibilities to attend most of our son's games. When the Big Green men's team came to town to play the Gophers, he was in the stands cheering for Dartmouth. As a grandpa, his favorite night out was Tommy's game followed by a pizza party. Even in mid-stage Alzheimer's, he could join the family at the Xcel Center and watch the Minnesota Wild play. He didn't necessarily know which team was which or what the score was, but he seemed to enjoy the game anyway.

I was a hockey fan, too. Born in Kansas, I came to the great state of hockey at age nine. When I was in junior high school, our high school team went to the state tournament. Busloads of kids traveled to St. Paul to fill the stands. The atmosphere was electric with school pride. When I became an Edina High School cheerleader, I never missed a game. The hard-skating boys on the team were our heroes; they took us back to the state tournament again and again. Several of them went on to play college hockey.

Phil's college hockey experience was a source of great pride for his family. Dartmouth coach Eddie Jeremiah had actually come to the Roy home to recruit Phil. As a sophomore, Phil became a part of the 1960 All Ivy Championship Team. A forward on the third line, he was fast and a good shooter. News of his team's success and his prowess reached Minnesota. His mom made sure all her friends had copies of the newspaper clippings, one of which dubbed Phil "Dartmouth's Darling": he'd scored twice and made an assist against Harvard. Alice answered the phone for weeks, "Dartmouth's Darling's mother speaking." A neighbor was king of St. Paul's Winter Carnival; he knighted Phil as Sir Shoot and Score Some More. Just getting to know Phil and his family, I listened to these stories with bemusement. Phil clearly had heroic status in his tribe.

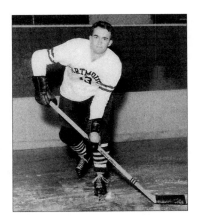

*Phil on the Dartmouth team*

In preparation for the fiftieth reunion, Dartmouth's All-American goalie, Tom Wahman, had submitted an entry for the team's memory book that included Phil. Rusty called Tom and told him about Phil's health problems. Tom forwarded the piece via email to me and followed with a phone call.

His story recalled Phil committing a cheap penalty near the end of a game where Dartmouth was already a man short. As the goalie, Tom had lost heart with the greatly advantaged opponents bearing down on him; he had let in the winning goal. He'd been mad at Phil for putting him in a tough position. Tom remembered his anger interfering with his full defensive concentration.

The second part of Tom's memory piece took place decades later. Phil was a doctor at Bethesda Hospital in St. Paul. When he noted the Wahman name on a patient's door, Phil had stopped and introduced himself, asking the woman if she had a son named Tom who played hockey at Dartmouth. She said yes. After a lively chat about the Dartmouth years, Phil inquired about her health. Her problem was as yet undiagnosed. Phil asked if he could examine her abdomen and discovered a hard tumor the size of a grapefruit. Tom credited Phil with saving his mom's life, though Phil did not perform the surgery and the tumor was benign. In any case, Tom was hugely grateful to Phil for reaching out to his mom. Phil's part in the minor hockey incident was forever forgiven.

His story struck my heart because I could envision Phil's scrappiness and desperate penalty and because I knew Phil's wonderful physician touch. I sent the piece to all of our children as a reminder of their dad in his fullness.

In our phone conversation, Tom said he was coming to town in March. "Would it be reasonable to go see Phil?" he wondered. Phil was seldom communicative, but he still responded from the heart occasionally. I could not predict if he would be alert enough to respond. If Tom still wanted to go for himself, I offered to meet him in Rogers and go to Wellstead with him. I cautioned Tom that seeing the ravages of advancing Alzheimer's firsthand would be painful. I tried to let him off the hook, but he persisted.

I had no expectation that the meeting would mean anything to Phil, though I'd raised the Dartmouth hockey subject and shown him his skating photo the previous day in preparation. When Tom and I arrived at Wellstead, Phil was deeply asleep in his chair by the window. He looked ninety years old and puny. I knelt beside him, massaged his leg, rubbed his shoulder, spoke softly—all to arouse him gently. Tom sat on Phil's bed across the room patiently waiting. Phil's eyes would flutter but not stay open. After fifteen minutes or more, I said, "Phil, you have a visitor, Tom Wahman, from Dartmouth." Nothing. Tom came forward and sat beside Phil, speaking softly. Tom and I kept the conversation going. Tom had brought his antique hockey mask that looked like the contraption used to muzzle the serial killer in *The Silence of the Lambs*. He didn't want to scare Phil by putting it on, but it was an object of possible interest. Phil paid no attention.

Tom had his own car and could have excused himself at any time, but he persevered. He helped me lift Phil to a standing position, and we three proceeded to the lunch table. Phil was not interested in eating. The macaroni and cheese drew his clenched jaw. I retrieved a container of applesauce from the refrigerator; it was a winner. Phil began to brighten. I started over, "Phil, isn't it great to see Tom Wahman again!" Tom presented his hockey mask as a prompt. I brought out Phil's Dartmouth rugby shirt from his closet and danced the hanger before him. I asked Tom if there were a familiar Dartmouth song other than the infamous "Dartmouth's in Town Again, Run Girls Run." Phil was watching us with more interest. Then Tom sang the alma mater.

The atmosphere turned festive. Tom's clear singing voice stirred Phil's attention. Tom laughed at the lyric about granite in their muscles and their brains. He said his wife teased him that the words sounded as if they were all blockheads. His easy manner was beginning to draw Phil out. Phil said some words, not sentences, nothing with meaning. Still, we were all having a lovely time. Then Phil surprised us by saying, "Wahman." Tom had scored a rare connection!

Tom and I held Phil's arms and walked slowly around the memory care unit together. At last we settled Phil in his leather chair. He was exhausted. Tom said his good-bye. I accompanied him to the locked exit and gave him the code for the courtyard. We hugged in a grateful thank-you to each other. Tears glistened in our eyes. Together, we had awakened Phil's spirit.

Over the course of 2009, team members continued to encourage me to come to their February 2010 reunion. I was ambivalent about accepting their kind invitations to Hanover, feeling awkward and not really knowing anyone. Finally, a buried urge to represent Phil pushed me forward. Our daughter Jena, Dartmouth class of 1988, agreed to accompany me back to Hanover for the celebration. Cherished mother-daughter time and learning more about Phil created a win-win opportunity.

At the reunion headquarters, a roar of welcome greeted each arrival. Most of the guys had not seen each other in years. As Rusty was welcoming us, Tom came up behind me and covered my eyes with his hands. Like a little kid, he said, "I bet you don't know who this is." Of course I recognized his voice. Everyone was giddy, including the spouses, who seemed to catch the team fever.

Over the two days the players' stories drew Jena and me into Phil's youth and helped to bring the team back together. The first night in the lounge at Thompson Arena, most exchanges were one-on-one. One fellow told me how strong Phil was. Another guy remembered that he and Phil shared being quieter, more serious than others. That was a sweet surprise. Still another player said that Phil was such a gentleman. To a person, they said what a pleasure it had been to be on the team with Phil because he was fun and hardworking.

The formal luncheon banquet was held at the Hanover Inn. Rusty had set the roster of speakers into allotted time slots. Speaking from the heart, no presenter bothered with his notes or kept to the schedule. Despite unfulfilled promises of a bathroom break, no one in the audience left. A momentous, outpouring of treasured memories and tributes filled the room.

Their former athletic director sang the team's praises and described what they would have been up against in today's much bigger players, with muscles honed in the new weight room. Phil's teammates felt they would have handled such giants because of their faith in Coach Jeremiah. His messages, "Give the opponents your sneaky, wily look," and "Keep your eyes up and never give up fighting," had empowered them to many hard-fought victories.

I, too, was on the roster. I held aloft Phil's hockey photo, lovingly given to me so long ago. I admitted that Phil's Dartmouth Darling performance against Harvard was a family legend that I'd balanced in my mind with the thought, "One game doth not a hockey player make." I could see now that their golden time together had informed their lives. I told them that though Phil was never a man of reflection, I knew his love of the game, recalling how carefully he'd chosen North Star season tickets behind the goal so he could show me how the plays developed. Even now, I told them, I would intone the announcer's cry, "Let's play hockey!" to try to engage Phil in an occasional TV game. I vowed to take his new fiftieth reunion hat to him and share by virtue of my enthusiasm the wonderful experience I'd had.

As the group broke up, many folks thanked me for being willing to speak. They wanted Phil's piece in their collective quilt of experience. They had honored several deceased teammates and embraced a teammate with schizophrenia who was able to attend with his sister. John had spent ten years lost to his family, living in a car and flophouses. Recently found and somewhat rehabilitated, he didn't say much, wore two hats on top of each other, looked ten years older than his brethren, but nonetheless belonged. What a team!

Redressing Phil in smelly college hockey garb allowed my imagination to recapture some of my husband's vigor. From the beginning, I understood his competitive spirit and valued his effort to do his best. During many years of marriage, we clashed occasionally when we forgot we were on the same team. Oddly, Alzheimer's had given us a final chance to practice teamwork and to be glad for one another's best effort.

The players' genuine affection for each other fifty years later would have meant a lot to Phil. Instead, I was the beneficiary. I loved being in the company of those Dartmouth men, who valued their privilege of playing hockey. Their fond memories were seasoned with teasing and laughing at themselves. I was glad, too, for Jena to hear the stories of her dad as a young man. As we were losing Phil, we gained a wonderful, new chapter of his life from a time before either of us knew him.

Phil was much more than we could ever really know. Loving him, I gave thanks for what I did know of him: his strengths, his imperfections, his lightness of touch, his endurance, and his love.

## CHAPTER 17

# Loving

Jena and I drove dry roads back to Boston after the reunion in Hanover. The following day, snow fell heavily. Aboard my departure plane, I sat on the tarmac for two hours, as the pilot tried to time our departure amid repeated deicings, refueling, and forays to the takeoff strip suddenly blocked by snowplows. Stuck and challenged, I wondered if Phil felt his own helplessness as staff pushed his wheelchair to meals or slid the transfer belt around his torso to support him out of his chair and into the bathroom.

Once home I spent the next three days trying to reawaken our togetherness. Seated in a church service when I arrived at the nursing home, Phil was asleep. We shuffled back to his room with me holding onto his transfer belt. When he was comfortable in his recliner, I presented his new Dartmouth cap. I put it on his head. He took it off, perhaps not knowing what to make of it. On and off it went several times. He scrunched it in his iron grip as I recounted my time in Hanover. My enthusiasm for his team drew no connection to Dartmouth, to the hat, or to me. The next day I arrived for lunch and fed him. I might just as well have been an aide. With coaxing he opened his mouth, but my pleasantries elicited no positive spark. The third day, coming into his room, I turned off his TV to redirect his attention to us and still drew no smiles. Tired, and sadly aware that I was doing "seat" time more than connecting, I returned home to a cup of tea and the newspaper.

On that Friday my childhood friend Joanna joined me at the river for an overnight. Her husband, Paul, had died six months earlier after a short battle with cancer. We hoped to find comfort in one another. Her city boots with leather soles made my idea to tromp the river impractical. Setting out arm in arm down the middle of my plowed country road, we trusted our companionship to warm our loneliness. I cooked. We paid brief attention to David Brooks and Mark Shields on the *NewsHour*. We were our own informants, not on matters of state or world, but on existential matters of our personal reality.

Life on our own was not what we wanted or expected at this stage of our lives, but it was what we had. We agreed that our strong relationships with our children fed our well-being. We were both fortunate that our children invited us into their lives, knowing their challenges were not ours to solve nor their triumphs ours to claim. It was the loving connection with them that elevated our spirits.

Mostly we focused on ourselves. Jo admitted a meltdown, overwhelmed with the paperwork and dogged details of Paul's estate and financial matters he'd always been in charge of. Collapsed in her reading chair, she'd succumbed to a flood of tears with the cat perched on her heaving chest. Like me she could learn to do the work and get help for it, but its needing to be done was the stark reminder of our being on our own.

Our fiftieth high school reunion was taking place in September. Emails from classmates were flying back and forth as the planning proceeded. I told Jo about studying the Enneagram at my church retreat with a former colleague of our classmate David, who taught the Enneagram personality system in Europe. I reconnected my teacher to David via email and was astounded by David's reply to me, enclosing a poem he'd just written after a powerful dream of our adolescent days as a teenage couple. Feeling like that young girl for a moment awakened parts of me that had been dormant for a long time. The poem refreshed my own sense of the loveliness of longing. Pushing back my desk chair and staring happily out the window, I felt light and warmly wondrous. It was safe for me to confess to Jo that I had kept the secret poem and the sad fact that I'd given up on physical attraction to Phil in our tired circumstance. It was private, but I knew Jo would keep it safe.

Together we visited Phil the next morning. He was surprisingly alert at the breakfast table, where we joined him. Jo's experience with her sister Linda's Alzheimer's made her transition into Phil's world quite natural. Her smiles, banter, and laughter enlivened the table. Phil ate well, and then we three set out on a walk around the unit. Phil held tightly to both Jo's and my arms. Jo sang in her lovely voice. Phil spontaneously offered his duck call, a sure sign that he was having a fine time. My New Year's Eve wish that Phil would continue to find things in his life to make him smile was fulfilled.

Later that week I called to check in with Abby. Holding back tears, she said that the doctors had told her sister-in-law Katy that there was no more they could do for her. Her death from cancer was imminent. Katy had been a valiant fighter with a large, loving family squarely in her corner. Letting Katy go was a painful final step that none of them wanted or knew how to do. I ached for Katy's husband, seven children, and many grandchildren. I knew Abby and her husband, Ken, would give counsel and strength, but they were heartbroken, too. The price of their loving was high indeed.

I'd spent the previous Thanksgiving with Abby and Ken's family, including Katy. As we went around the table saying what we were thankful for, Katy had said she was actually grateful for her cancer. "My friends and family have given me so much love during this time. We've all been so present to each other. I'm overwhelmingly glad to feel the depth of our bonds." Her capacity to appreciate the goodness in her life was big to begin with, but it had actually grown.

Thinking of Phil, I was glad he did not have to suffer the physical pain that Katy endured. But I was also sorry for him. His loss of capacity made him seemingly incapable of appreciating the love bestowed on him. The doctors could not do anything for him, and neither could I. Sadness hung on my shoulders like a heavy winter coat.

Undone by Katy's news, Abby took the time to send me an affirming email: "Have I told you lately that I find you remarkable? How are you so able to move, to glide, from one important and intense issue or arena to the next, giving each full measure?" Abby's sense that I was moving with grace, actually gliding, reminded me to be grateful for my own good health. I knew that I bounced and lurched many times, but gliding was there too. Such feedback from my dear friend meant a lot to me. It helped me to appreciate myself and the God-given strength that propelled me.

The unexpectedly warm weather in March 2010 made me eager for spring and taking Phil outside once again. He'd always been an outdoor guy. Being shut in for the winter had been a long haul, restricting us to carpeted hallways—even if the handrails were a godsend for his off-balance gait.

When the ice went out of the St. Croix River and leaf buds began to pop, I decided to venture out with Phil. I bundled him up and transferred him to a wheelchair to claim the sunshine. At the pond I pointed out the duck pairs and made quacking sounds, but Phil didn't relate to the scene or my antics. Two squawky geese on the path did call him to attention. For some reason I'd brought Mariah along on a leash. We were all in a state of agitation, so I turned us around and headed back. Mariah ran in front and then behind, twisting her slack leash in the wheels of the chair as I pushed Phil up the incline toward the building. I was in a sweat before we got inside. When I helped Phil out of his coat back in his room, his hands were ice cold.

I admitted to Heidi that I'd made our first outing of the season too complicated. The next day she carefully walked Phil to the elevator and out into the interior courtyard so they could sit in the sun. "Mom, Dad seemed really lighthearted," she reported. Might spring perk Phil up? I hoped so. She and I continued to get Phil outside for fresh air. Without Mariah, I returned us to the duck pond. With the wheelchair brake locked and me sitting next to him on the park bench, Phil seemed to enjoy himself.

Pleasant weather persisted. By the end of April Heidi wondered aloud, "I think this time last year Dad may have been overmedicated." Phil's seizures during the winter of 2008–2009 had traumatized him and us. In hindsight, the pharmacological response may have been excessive. We couldn't be sure. After Phil's move to Boutwells Landing, Dr. Holm weaned him off the antiseizure meds. With the increased staffing ratio, the improved food, our easy access, and fewer drugs, Phil seemed to be at least on a plateau physically.

Beth had planned another international adventure and again invited me to join her family. In May we went to China. The day before I left I had a very tender visit with Phil. His eyes were bright, his demeanor quiet and relaxed. I fed him his favorite raspberries, massaged his hands with cream, clipped his fingernails, sat with him for lunch, and supported him in a walk inside. I was sorry that he could not go on the kind of adventure that I would soon have. I also felt a surge of gladness for our many years together. I recounted some of our old adventures to him. Phil stared at my teary eyes and nodded his head, as if to affirm my tales and feelings. He was paying attention as best he could. In that precious moment I felt we were together, tuned in our own ways.

"Go have fun, Mom," Heidi blessed me at departure. Brief getaways had been a boon to my mental health in recent years, but this was a full-fledged vacation. I pulled the plug on responsibility for two weeks. How fortunate both Phil and I were to have Heidi's loving support and the professional team at Boutwells Landing!

China was amazing in size, in number of people, in antiquities, and in its modernity. Cait's blonde hair drew more picture taking from the locals than the giant pandas in the Beijing Zoo. The little girls ran up the steps of the Great Wall effortlessly, while I paused often to catch my breath and drink in the hillsides covered with blooming cherry trees. "Go ahead," I encouraged the young family. Being halfway around the world from home leaning against the historic parapet, I could scarcely take in all the changes in our world and my small life. My knee hurt, too.

In Xian the terra-cotta warriors stretched my imagination. The sheer size of the underground army of unique figures, which date back to 600 CE, defies understanding of how the craftsmen created them. The emperor's belief that they would protect his spirit in the afterlife certainly seemed foreign. My own belief in resurrection didn't require such elaborate physical preparations. My plan was to have dear Phil cremated and buried in the Garth (the inner courtyard) at House of Hope Church.

On our last day in Hong Kong, Oliver left on business. Beth and I took the girls to Hong Kong Disney as promised. Beth used the hotel Internet connection to review the timetable of all events and led us in an exciting and efficient sequence of rides, shows, and eating that allowed air-conditioned reprieve from a hot, sunny day. My role was to save a spot in line, find a Wet Wipe, and have fun myself. The Chinese version of Disney was spectacular, featuring their own fine artists with the traditional characters unchanged. Cinderella was Cinderella. The Lion King performance with enormous animal floats and lively dancers coming into the audience swept all of us into the story, despite the language difference.

Returning to Boutwells Landing, I reentered Phil's quiet world. He was sleepy, which was how Heidi had often found him in my absence. Maybe he was winding down. I didn't selfishly want to wind him up if that was counter to his own stage of withdrawal. Finally, one day, he was awake. I cozied up to him on my folding chair, offered sips of cold grape juice, held his cold hand, looked him in the eyes, grinned encouragingly, chattered some, and allowed silences. I was glad to be back together.

I wanted Phil to have loving attention and to feel cared about. This desire still stood after nearly four years of residential care. In my view excellent staff could do only so much, even though they were more important to his daily, physical well-being than I was. Phil was a respected resident. To me, he was also a beloved husband, father, and grandfather. I wanted him to know that in any way possible.

On the other hand, sometimes I honestly dreaded seeing him. Seeing his decline and experiencing our squashed, lopsided life wore on me. I relied on my feet to carry me automatically into the building and my heavy heart to come along obediently.

When I happily welcomed Mother back for the summer, she was a bit quick to say, "You are a Pollyanna. Phil doesn't really know you." How she came to her conclusion was not clear. "Phil's knowing me is not a matter for debate, Mother," I told her. I felt he knew me even though he was fading away. Such knowing was not a matter of calling my name or remembering our forty-six years together. It was a matter of trusted touch, comfortable presence, responsive smile, and lack of account. Old hurts and joys were set aside, but brief moments of new gladness had not entirely dimmed.

Jena, Max, and Mimi came to Minnesota for the Fourth again. Phil's seventieth birthday loomed. What could the family do to celebrate with him? Planning an occasion was senseless. Phil was only present when he was present, which could not be predicted for a specified time on a certain date. Late one afternoon on a solo visit to Phil, I found him very awake. Hoping he would stay alert, I called home and rallied the troops to come quick.

Heidi, Jena, Mother, and six grandchildren appeared with a chocolate ice cream cake from Dairy Queen and birthday hats. Phil didn't even have to get out of his recliner. We brought extra chairs into his room; grandson Tom sat in Phil's wheelchair. We sang and cut the cake. Jena and Heidi took turns spooning the ice cream into Phil's eager mouth. He even laughed out loud. We were all touched. I snapped a joyous picture for our Christmas card collage. I wanted friends to see Phil having fun.

Shortly thereafter Max, Mimi, Walter (Heidi's son), and I left on a carefully planned trip on the Empire Builder to see their Uncle Chris in Montana. In preparation for the trip, Walt and I went to Mitchell's Fly Shop in Lake Elmo. We hoped to do some fly-fishing and needed to check our fishing equipment so we'd be ready. We waited our turn in the small shop, looking at the displays and mounted fish on the wall. The proprietor concluded his business with the only other customer and turned to us, "How may I help you?"

I began to explain that Walt and I were going out West where my husband and I used to fish and burst into tears. The rush of emotion was unexpected. Grief ambushed me! I stopped my words, blinked back my tears, and muttered an apology. The sensitive fellow offered, "You needn't be sorry." I returned, "Well, I'm not sorry to weep. But the sudden feeling caught me off guard. My Phil used to come to this shop to tie flies. We loved to fish together and had wonderful times." Walter stood at my side undaunted, allowing this difficult moment to pass. When he sensed we were back on track, he presented his equipment and showed the flies that he'd tied himself.

Watching my young fisherman reminded me happily of his grandpa. The reel that I'd saved was junk, so I bought a new, smoothly operating

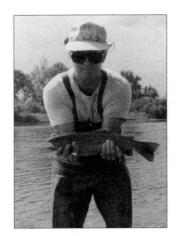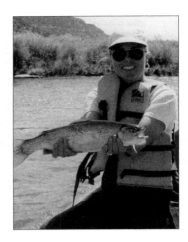

*Phil and me with our catch from the Bow River, 1990s*

one with fresh line and tippet. Waiting for its setup on Phil's Powell rod, I regained composure, warmed by the prospect of our upcoming adventure.

I would never be able to recreate my fly-fishing days with Phil except in memory. They represented the best in our relationship, companionable time spent out of doors, away from work demands, and full of good humor. We often hired guides on those precious days to assure fruitful fishing and more often to assist me. One old hand tried to improve my technique. The wrist motion between eleven and one o'clock that loads the line did not come easily to me. "Barbara, you are not driving a Conestoga wagon!" he observed wryly. I started to laugh and looked down. There, swimming around my waders, trout were eating the food I'd kicked up from the streambed. Amid such abundance, I could have scooped one up with my net. Phil was a natural fisherman, like Robert Redford in *A River Runs Through It*. His delivery stretched effortlessly and accurately to distant targets. He was beautiful to watch. Luckily for me, not all streams had required long casts.

On this new trip to Montana Chris was anxious to show us the natural marvels in Glacier National Park. At Logan Pass he hoped to take me on an alpine walk to see many wildflowers. Instead snowfields covered the low meadows. Walt commandeered a cardboard box from the gift shop and attempted some sledding. When he spotted some big-horn sheep resting in the snow, he ventured too close to them with my camera and received a reprimand from a park ranger. His self-invented fun and unconcern for boundaries reminded me of Phil. Chris patiently gathered us up and shepherded us on our way. He reminded me a bit of myself. He was a wonderful host.

At the end of July Beth's family returned to Minnesota. Cait and Imogen were excited to visit Grandpa and his playground. To minimize commotion, I suggested Beth and the girls go ahead to the playground while I went upstairs to collect Grandpa. The girls were so dear with him, giving hugs and calling to him, "Watch this!" They paid no attention to Phil's deficits. He was simply Grandpa. Phil sat passively in his wheelchair, putting up no resistance as they snitched treats from his box of Junior Mints. Happiness reigned.

Over the course of their month's stay, there were many such visits to Boutwells Landing. I continued to go on my own, too. I needed staff assistance to transfer Phil to his wheelchair for the outdoor times. Indoors I always tried to walk with Phil. I asked staff to keep up a walking routine, thinking that mobility was good for him both physically and emotionally. Phil had never been a sitter in his whole life, and I wanted him to be able to move. For safety he wore a transfer belt. Unfortunately his legs buckled more and more frequently, so the nursing home required two staff to walk with Phil. Finding two available staff at the same time was not easy. With his sleepiness and staff demands, Phil didn't often have chances to walk. Hardheaded, I took him by myself.

The summer ended with a priceless gift from Cait to me. I loved having her as my roommate and kept a twin mattress on my bedroom floor for her. Our deal was that she couldn't wake me up until six thirty a.m. On the last morning, she snuggled into my big bed with me and said, "Oh, Gigi, I wish it was yesterday so I could have one more day with you!" Her tenderness and loving message innocently expressed gave me unforgettable and immeasurable joy. The loss of Phil's wholeness cast no shadow.

Soon Chris and his girlfriend, Amber, came home over Labor Day. I managed to create a picnic to include Heidi's family. I'd intended to go see Phil early, but I ended up waving to his building and driving straight home from the grocery store. Amber and Chris had gone off on a walk. Mother wanted to know why I was home earlier than expected. "It's not like you *not* to go see Phil. Do you feel all right?" she mothered me. What I felt was that I'd like to be walking with Chris, not defending my health. I put away the groceries and set out on a walk by myself. I had to accept that I could not do all the things I wanted to do. I needed to calm down. Walking alone, I admitted to myself that spending time with Phil was harder and harder. I didn't feel as if I had much to give him. I hated feeling useless, and I was tired of feeling sad. There was no way to escape either feeling.

Back in the kitchen, family life resumed. Mother shucked the corn and tasted the potato salad for seasoning. Amber chopped the vegetables, while Chris set the table. Heidi's daughter Jane, who was ten, brought dessert. Heidi's other daughter, Susan, who was nine, and her mother performed gymnastic feats on the lawn. I timed foot races around the path through my prairie grasses. We were at ease hanging out and sharing a meal.

Mid-September was Phil's annual checkup with Dr. Holm. He'd not ridden in a car since the previous year's checkup. Heidi helped with all the transfers between car and wheelchair. Essentially there was nothing new. In Dr. Holm's words, "Phil is frail but healthy. He's had very good care. Still, if something were to assault his body, he wouldn't have much strength to fight back." It was lousy to know that Phil's life was both precarious and likely to go on in an even more debilitated state.

Switching to my fiftieth high school reunion seemed odd. Joanna and I decided to be each other's date because we had no partners. I stayed with her in Minneapolis so I wouldn't have to drive so far for the three days of events. The informal buffet, get-reacquainted party on Friday night was fun, but I dreaded the more formal cocktail, dinner, and dancing gathering on Saturday. As much as I loved Joanna, I had no intention of dancing with her. The party would be held at Interlachen Country Club, where Phil and I had enjoyed our wedding reception. I tried to remind myself that this party was not about me and to get over myself.

In the whirl of friendly classmates, Joanna and I got separated during cocktail hour but reconnoitered at a table by the band for dinner. Classmate Franz had hired the Rockin' Hollywoods to liven up the evening. He joined in their sets wearing a silver jacket and sunglasses, playing guitar. The rock-and-roll music transported all of us to our teenage sock-hop era. When one of my favorite fellows grabbed my hand and led me to the dance floor, I was a kid again. How lucky we'd been to belong to this great class of 1960.

My childhood boyfriend David came all the way from Italy. We were amused and bemused to find ourselves on the dance floor after fifty years. Whatever moves we made, our eyes were pretty much locked. I felt as if I might fall into that sweet gaze. Whether our connection was old or new, situational or continual, it was strong. During our final dance, a slow one to "Unchained Melody," David embraced me and closed his eyes. We were not clumsy kids. It felt wonderful to be held, to be cherished, to feel beautiful, and to let myself go.

Joanna and I left by eleven, since we had responsibilities during the memorial service the next morning. Up early, we were excited and ready to do our parts. Jo was to lead a trio of singers, and I was to give a reflection on loss. The singers began the service with "It's a Beautiful World." The last of several speakers, I recited Robert Frost's poem "Nothing Gold Can Stay" and spoke of the impermanence in life that makes most of us uneasy. "But," I said,

> it gives us all the more reason to celebrate in the here and now. The good news of love and friendship and freedom gives us great cause. Who has a new grandchild? Who has a dear friend? Who wants to vote in 2012? Who has a new calling? Who is eager to travel? Who has a home, maybe even without a mortgage? Who has a new hip, a hearing aide, a stent? Who has a quiet place to restore his or her spirit? Most importantly, who feels loved by a partner, a child, a friend, or yet a parent? . . .
>
> Good fortune abounds! Even when times are personally tough, situations sad, or worries many, we know we've been blessed. We give thanks for the lives of our deceased classmates, for our own

lives, and for the lives of all the men and women who defend freedom and extend hands of compassion to the downtrodden. Our glad hearts sing!

Joanna's trio immediately broke into "Those Were the Days," which erupted into a conga line of 160 dancing souls singing, "La la la la la," as we went inside to eat.

David and I sat together to enjoy the last hour of the reunion. On the back of our memorial program, Mary Oliver's poem "Snow Geese" captured our experience perfectly. David was my snow goose who would fly on. To have seen and appreciated him was a lovely treasure.

Returning to Phil after the emotionally charged weekend, I found him awake and asked him gently, "Do you feel my love?" By luck or by soulful spark, he broke into a smile. I had loved him as best I could for a long time. Going through the trials of Alzheimer's had not been easy for either of us. If Phil had been able to ask me the same question, I was unsure of my response. Mostly, I remembered his love. Poor darling, he could not remember anything.

# CHAPTER 18

# Pulling Teeth

In the gloomy, dark days of late 2010 I ordered Phil's teeth pulled. His teeth grinding and compromised dental hygiene had left stumps jagged to his tongue and busy finger. Neither of us could see into his mouth, which he no longer opened on command. My imagination and fear, however, slipped through his flaccid lips and encountered stalactites of decay and swollen, infected gums. I reasoned with myself, if a tooth is not there, it cannot ache. I was desperate to ward off the possibility of Phil being in physical pain.

My helpless, seventy-year-old husband with his blue Paul Newman eyes wasn't eating well again. More weight loss emphasized his chiseled chin and cheekbones. "In sickness and health," we had pledged long ago. Alzheimer's had called on that pledge ten years earlier. Since then, it had been eating away Phil's strength and personality. It had nearly devoured our life together. Now it demanded that I make yet another health care decision to protect Phil.

We had always been faithful to our six-month dental checkups. After Phil's diagnosis, I maintained the routine for two reasons. First, I valued oral health. And, second, our trip to the dental office had felt normal, even as Alzheimer's progressed. The receptionist, the hygienist, and the dentist were familiar faces and caring professionals. The office atmosphere was friendly and welcoming. Phil was still Phil in their eyes. They knew our situation; I didn't have to explain it.

Dr. Stratton was also a friend, a good golfer, and a blessed clown. On Monday afternoons, when Phil was still living at home, when usual play was suspended while the maintenance crew cared for our golf course, I would drive Phil to town to meet Glenn so they could play some holes at their own pace. The club pro sanctioned this weekly plan. Phil saw the arrangement as nothing out of the ordinary. His muscle memory meant he could still wallop the ball. Glenn didn't care if Phil chose to hit the wrong ball or took a long time to replace the cover on his club. They didn't keep score.

Alzheimer's added odd twists to their game. Standing on the tee box, Phil didn't remember how to aim for the green or where it was necessarily. Glenn would line him up and applaud his good shot. In the fairway, Phil would take out a tee and set up his ball for another big shot. As the distance to the green shortened, Glenn would quickly substitute Phil's wedge for the driver. If they chose to putt, the cup was often an irrelevant target. A joke and a laugh completed the hole most satisfactorily. Then it was time for a cart ride.

When Glenn himself retired, he made sure that we were comfortable with the new man who bought his practice. After Phil entered residential care, I continued to make the long-distance trip to the familiar dental office. Similarly to the way he used muscle memory in golf, Phil would walk into the office with his natural joie de vivre. Like church, there was an order to the service. We signed in, we sat down to wait our turn, we began with the hygienist, the dentist read the X-rays and examined the teeth, we were given new toothbrushes and perhaps another appointment for crown work, we paid, we had a cordial time, and we were done in an hour. We belonged to the practice.

Eventually, Phil could no longer care for his teeth himself. He did not like his noisy electric toothbrush any more; he resisted the initial offers of oral care by assisted living staff at Wellstead. Toothpaste became a puzzlement to him; he smeared his tube's contents on the bathroom wall. A nonelectric toothbrush was instituted and, together with the toothpaste, stored in the staff room. I hoped his cooperation would come.

One day, when I tried to wipe a piece of food from one of Phil's lower front teeth, I discovered that the tooth itself was dark. The enamel was rubbery to my touch. Then, to my horror, the tooth broke off. The exposed remnant demanded attention. What was the condition of his teeth in general? I disguised my alarm for Phil's sake but immediately notified staff and called for an emergency dental appointment. Phil seemed unconcerned, not noticing the irregularity in his mouth right away.

The next day, Phil, Heidi, and I were gathered in the dental office. Heidi assumed a clinical eye and offered emotional support to both Phil and me. The hygienist had the gruesome task of cleaning Phil's mouth. In the familiar setting, with us gently and reassuringly holding his hands, he did not resist. X-rays showed rampant decay. Despite our love for the man, Heidi and I were repulsed by what we saw! Without flossing and careful brushing and plenty of water drinking, old food was stuck to his teeth in a gooey slime.

Soon Phil became agitated. He wanted up and out of the chair. The dentist could not consider attempting the complex process of setting a temporary cap on the broken tooth. He referred us to an oral surgeon, who could perhaps do the work under mild anesthesia.

Several days later, Heidi teamed with me again for the oral surgeon appointment, yet farther away. The trip represented an equilateral triangle with one-hour sides. She drove an hour to pick up her dad. I drove an hour to the surgeon's office so I could meet them at the front door. Heidi was to stay for the procedure and head home. I would drive Phil back and eventually return home myself.

As they drove up, I greeted them and helped Phil inside without incident. Heidi parked and joined us. We were on a family outing; Phil was relaxed and happy to be the center of attention for he knew not what. Prior to his procedure, a new X-ray was required. The request for him to stand still with his head resting against a metal plate so the film could be taken went unheeded. Phil assumed the correct position a dozen times but moved away again too quickly.

The oral surgeon came into the exam room to confer with our family. He was interested and full of kind advice, just the way Phil would have been in his professional days. He understood that Alzheimer's was in the room too. In the end, he recommended doing nothing surgically. He felt the tooth's dentin, the layer under the enamel, would protect the tooth as well as a rough-fitting temporary cap under the circumstances. Heidi and I were satisfied with the suggested approach of doing nothing, trusting the advice given and knowing no better solution.

We celebrated our unexpected extra time together by going out to lunch in a nearby strip mall. At his advanced disease stage, Phil had forgotten how to sit down automatically, but we finally settled at a table. The place was busy and noisy, not an easy atmosphere in which to relax. When we finished eating, I assured Heidi that I could handle things going forward and that she should hurry home in time for her children to arrive after school. I felt confident that I could handle getting Phil to our car, driving back to his care center, coaching him into the building, helping him find his room, and eventually making my way home through rush-hour traffic. I knew my duty, and I was up to it.

When Phil and I set out for the parking lot in the cold afternoon air, I guided him easily to our car and opened the passenger door. Then it occurred to me that he didn't know how to get into the car. Without Heidi or staff to assist, I was left to find a way to unlock our predicament on the spot. Fortunately, our crazy circumstance somehow struck me funny. Phil joined my laughter. I hugged him and decided to dance us around the car for as many approaches as it took to have him slip into the passenger seat without having to think. Around and around we circled until I finally said, "Phil, I'm cold. We better pop in." He did, and we left. The unexpected parking-lot dance was a beautiful gift. We'd had fun thanks to a broken tooth and grace.

After Phil moved to Boutwells Landing, he began grinding his teeth. He sounded like the old electric rock polisher our young kids used on the summer porch—only we couldn't unplug this machine. Slowly and over time, one tooth broke, and then another. His increased trips to the in-house hygienist simply could not stem the tide of decay. With the help of Ativan and more hand holding, Phil had allowed those checkups, but by the end of October 2010 six more teeth had cracked off rapidly. What to do?

Like Phil, I was a doer by nature. Now I was the doer for both of us. I tried to face difficulty before it became intolerable. I'd had to accept Phil's diagnosis, but I had been anxious to preserve his body and spirit,

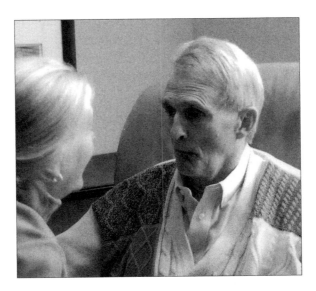

*Phil and me, Boutwells Landing, 2010*

if not his mind. Next Alzheimer's ravaged his physical self. I missed his off-balance gait. I used to be able to hold his arm and bear his weight as we circled his care unit. Now, unseen, I pushed him in a wheelchair whenever we left his room. Ambulation was gone.

I understood that I could not stop the crumbling of his teeth. Still, my desire to prevent the chance of pain from rampant infection continued. The attending physician at the nursing home said that Phil could endure mild sedation without further deterioration, so I directed the dentist to extract the rotten teeth a few at a time.

Phil was not a candidate for dentures. I worried that the substructure of his smile was being dismantled. Speechless, his smile had thanked and encouraged me along the way. It had signaled that he was okay and didn't feel scared. It had been his gift to me. I couldn't abide losing it.

I was undone by being in the dental operating theater for the first extractions. The sedation had not put Phil out completely. I didn't know whether he would feel pain during the procedure. He looked so vulnerable. My presence to hold his hand comforted neither of us. I called the clinical director on the nursing home floor upstairs to replace me. She could keep his hands safely out of the dentist's way. Unhappily, I took my place in the waiting room. A recurrent sense of loss weighed on my heart, my eyes closed, and my shoulders drooped. I felt useless, power-less, and deeply sad. My resilient, positive attitude vanished. I was too tired to rage against the senselessness of our puny reality. I was numb.

More extractions were to come. Phil could not anticipate his next loss, but he would be submitted to it. I posted the dental schedule in his room. There was no tooth fairy in his losing proposition—just inevitability.

# CHAPTER 19

# Saying Good-Bye

In January 2011 I had a vivid dream. In it I was driving a semitruck. On the flatbed trailer an aircraft was mounted sideways. The plane's nose and tail were perpendicular to the road and spilled out of my lane on both sides. Looking at the road ahead, I saw a bridge spanning the highway; it was much too low for my unusual load. Waking up with alarm, I mused, "What kind of a nut am I to be driving such an unwieldy load?"

I knew the load in that dream was not Alzheimer's alone. The image might have been a reminder once again for me to stop trying to do too much. I'd had a full house of four generations of family for Christmas week. A resurgence of community meetings had required my frequent attendance after the holidays. I really wanted to try memoir writing and had contacted a writing coach. Visiting Phil remained my priority in the mix. And to restore my own soul, I knew that I also needed to preserve some uncluttered time with no demands.

A mysterious force deep within me was calling me to wrestle with memoir. I sent the writing coach some samples from my journals before our first meeting, hoping that she could see that they would be a natural springboard to memoir writing. In the cover letter, I wrote that what I wanted to attempt would "NOT be about the science of disease or caregiving tips; it would be about our human response to inexplicable change, real loss, and brutal reality. At the same time, it would celebrate the dignity of life, the sustainability of spirit, and the beauty of the moment." On the phone I told her I needed a coach to challenge me, keep me on task, and offer real criticism. I didn't need someone to like me; I needed someone who would tell me the truth about my writing.

Phil was fading. The day before I was to meet the coach, I groaned inwardly. I had no real plan for my new writing, much less an initial attempt. After church and before going to the nursing home to see Phil, I decided to stop at Perkins for pancakes and to focus on my writing plan. I was dog-tired. Waiting for my order, I dug in my purse for a pen and paper. The only piece of paper was a small bank receipt. Thus equipped, I tried to think. I wrote down "teeth"; we were in the throes of Phil's desperate need for dental care. My food came. Between bites, I wrote other single, random words: river, boat, dogs, trips, hockey, trees. Food consumed, I left. Entering Phil's world at the care center, I shelved all other thoughts. Afterwards I don't remember what I did, but I know I showed up the next day at the coach's office with a crumpled bank receipt and nothing more.

She told me that journal writing was linear. If I wanted to grow my writing, I would need to go deeper and explore my feelings in revision after revision. My idea to cut and paste pieces from my journals was inadequate. I despaired at the thought of starting over. She also pointed out that if I were going to attempt memoir, then the story would have to be about me, not Phil. In recent years my life had seemingly and necessarily been all about Phil. I was not totally lost to myself, but I often had had to set myself aside in considering Phil's needs. Raking through the hubris and loving myself would be a big assignment. Who, indeed, was I? Who would I be on my own? How might I make peace with the difficulties in my life?

It was time to face myself. Maybe the load on that semi in my dream was a metaphor for the task at hand. I was at the wheel, I would exceed my narrow lane, and I would encounter barriers to my progress. The new writing was difficult. I immediately battled with my internal editor, assailing myself with more questions. How is this work meaningful to me or anyone else? What am I learning? Why am I spending time doing this? I wasn't comfortable feeling so self-absorbed. I goaded myself: "What you really need is physical exercise!"

On gray, wintry mornings I lay in bed at first light watching snow fall against the cedars outside my sliding door. Memories consumed me, jostling each other for position in the story. Conscious and subconscious recollections awakened my sense of self. Paying attention, I felt tender and full and unhurried.

Up the road at Boutwells Landing Phil was changing too. Staff had to use a lift to swing him from bed, to bath, to recliner, to wheelchair. Phil didn't seem to mind. He was seldom resident in his own ragdoll body.

One day I was late in visiting him. The attendant was feeding him pureed peas and mashed potatoes, both of which were smeared on his pants. I was delighted to see his bright eyes and messy grin at my approach. I had brought myself a sandwich so I could join the evening meal. The attendant and I chatted while they finished and I ate. After wheeling Phil back to his room, I gently washed his face and hands with a soapy washcloth. He liked the warmth. I removed the chocolate pudding dessert drool. Then, five minutes later, there it was again. And again. I gave lots of face washes.

Several days later one of the associate pastors from our church came to the nursing home to see us. Phil was seated in a new, high-backed wheelchair at the breakfast table, hair combed and cleanly shaven. He didn't see us come in, so I took the pastor into Phil's room for a private chat. He wanted to know the background story of our situation. I poured forth information like a well-used pitcher, apologizing a bit for the matter-of-fact outline. I told him, "We've been on this journey for a long time. I'm resigned to its being what it is." I retrieved Phil's book about his life, and we joined him at the breakfast table.

Together we went over the pictures of family, career, interests, and our homes on the St. Croix River. Phil's eyes seemed to follow our voices and the turning pages; he actually tried to speak. I hoped he recognized himself somehow. Before leaving, the pastor offered a prayer for us. I was both uncomfortable and touched by his plea on my behalf. I didn't like others to notice or remind me of my vulnerability. In my mind, Phil was the vulnerable one.

I stayed for lunch. The pumpkin soup smelled good. When I requested fresh fruit too, the aide said she would have some pureed. I wanted Phil to have nutrition, flavor, and texture. I assured her I would cut up the pieces into small bits. Phil did, in fact, have a coughing spasm with one of the mandarin oranges. So I was reminded that his new special diet was for a reason. Nevertheless, at his subsequent care conference, I signed a waiver so that I could give him finely chopped fruit occasionally. I didn't want to think of him devoid of all pleasure.

On Wednesday, January 26, I drove into town for lunch with Anne Simpson and circled back to visit Phil. He was deeply asleep. I turned on soft music, held his hands, and waited for him to come around. After an hour, I left, unworried. Phil's sleepiness was not unusual.

The next day I attended a Wilder Foundation board meeting early and joined Phil for lunch. He was groggy and without appetite, again not totally unusual. I got him to take a few tiny bites of his pureed meal, but he had difficulty swallowing. When he opened his mouth, I could see remaining food collected there. I didn't want to force food, so I pushed him away from the table. In his room, I prepared warm washcloths to clean him up. Food continuously drizzled from the corners of his mouth. He did not register the warmth or my presence. I sat in his recliner and pulled his wheelchair close to me.

Sitting in his padded chair, he was higher than I was, which allowed his bent head to look down at me. I massaged his calves with lotion for a long time, and he seemed to brighten. I sang and smiled at him and was rewarded by his smile. When the aides came in to take him to the bathroom, I kissed him good-bye and left. They would settle Phil into his recliner with a cozy blanket for a nap.

On Friday I went to a birthday luncheon and met with my writing coach before heading back to Boutwells Landing. I arrived in time for Phil's five p.m. supper. Seated at his usual table, he again was asleep. My effort to stir him and offer sustenance was futile. Real alarm bells finally sounded in my head.

Again, we left the table and returned to the quiet of his room. When the aides came to ready him for bed, I ached looking at his scrawny body suspended from the E-Z Lift. I called Heidi to download the brutal reality of her dad's withered, unresponsive state.

Heidi awakened on Saturday morning at five a.m. thinking about her dad. She emailed her siblings and me with a heartfelt, medical warning that if Phil could not eat, his body would shut down rather rapidly. I arrived at Boutwells at breakfast time and spent all day with Phil. He was dressed, sitting in his recliner without affect or appetite. We did not bother to go to the dining room. Heidi appeared for a face-to-face assessment at suppertime. I took a brief break and went to Kowalski's to get us some soup. While we ate, I told her that Phil had been reweighed and was down ten pounds that week and I'd ordered hospice, which could not start until Tuesday. "Oh, Mom," she concurred.

When Phil was settled in bed for the night, I went home to sleep. He did not seem in any pain or anxiety. My thoughts turned to when the children should come. No one knew how long dying would take. Perhaps a week? Beth made immediate reservations to arrive Thursday. Jena called to say she had reservations to come Monday night. Beth switched her reservations to Tuesday. Chris was standing by. Ever faithful, Heidi was close by, albeit working and caring for her large family.

Sunday morning was very cold. A glorious cock pheasant strutted across the road in front of the car on my way to Phil. I thought how much it reminded me of him and how much he would have enjoyed seeing it. I braked the car and watched until he disappeared into the brush. With shining feathers, he took his time, allowing me to appreciate his beauty. I'd not seen a pheasant on our street in years. This sudden, magnificent specimen enthralled me. He seemed to glow in the sunlight. Phil could not absorb my rapturous tale, but I knew that pheasant and he were one.

At Boutwells, staff asked if I wanted them to dress Phil and put him in his chair. We agreed that he'd be more comfortable in his bed. While they were freshening him up, I broke down. He was a skeleton. The scientific reality of the body shutting down was small compared to my realization that he was soon done.

Snow was eddying in the corner by his third-story window. It was snowing up! Was it a message from Phil? Watching the updraft, I felt a surge of love for Phil and all his unique difference. Looking at him, I knew he was blowing away, too. I called Heidi. "It's happening," I whispered. Before she joined me at the nursing home, I reached our out-of-town children and wept, "Come now."

I called church to alert our pastor, David Van Dyke, that Phil was dying. By pure luck he was in his office after the Sunday morning service and picked up the phone. He promised to join us by two p.m. All I could do was to sit beside Phil and hold his hand, that precious hand that I'd squeezed in the pain of childbirth, in the sweetness of walking side by side, in the acknowledgment of mutual understanding, in the assurance of presence, and in the tenderness of coming sleep.

Heidi arrived and crawled onto the bed beside her dad, stroking his face and speaking softly to him. His breath rattled; his expression remained frozen. As a trio, we formed a sculpture of death and devotion. Phil's eyes fluttered only once on hearing the surprise voice of dear friend Joanna. With her signature, fresh-baked *kringler* in hand, she sang into the room, "Oh, Philemon, I love you so much." Her few minutes with us left a glow of friendship. When David came, he brought the comfort of prayer and readiness to tend our whole family. Nestled between the wall and Phil, Heidi never left her dad's side during the brief visits. I managed only to stand to accept embraces. Stillness and quiet prevailed. The nursing staff arranged for end-of-life medications to ease Phil's breathing. It was obvious that hospice on Tuesday would be too late.

Still holding his hand, I finally used my cell phone to call Abby, who was away in California, and Phil's sisters. If Phil could hear my soft voice in these tender conversations, then, too, I hoped he might sense my love and acceptance.

By dinnertime, first Chris arrived, and then Jena. Heidi demonstrated a natural ease in the face of death, both matter-of-fact and loving. She moved Phil's bed perpendicular to the wall to give each of her siblings space to take one of his hands. I shifted to massaging his feet. When staff came to reposition Phil's limp body, Heidi and I stepped out of the room briefly. Then came the whispered alarm, "Dad's stopped breathing." Heidi explained that stopping and restarting was to be expected. Sure enough, Phil resumed his breaths, and the vigil continued. Heidi left to bring back some supper.

The repeated disappearance of Phil's breath, our urgent listening for its return, and the shock of its sudden reappearance—all took me back to our long-ago hikes as a young family. The children and I reminisced about Phil's days as a playful troll in the woods, leaping out from behind trees to surprise us. In the gravity of the moment, we felt the joy of loving our Silly Philly.

Beth arrived moments after Phil's final breath just before midnight. Jena had put her ear to Phil's chest; his heartbeat was no more. I went downstairs to unlock the nursing home door and rode the elevator up to Phil's room with her. "Did I make it, Mom?" "Almost," I said softly. Phil's spirit had ascended, but his warm body allowed Beth to touch and say her farewell to his earthly presence.

On the drive home from Boutwells Landing, gigantic snowflakes were falling fast. Our lone car headlights illuminated pristine, white farm fields. No tire tracks marred the almost indistinguishable roadway. Tired and transfixed, we drove slowly into our new life without Phil.

# CHAPTER 20

## Celebrating and Grieving

In the morning six-year-old Caitlyn woke me up by tickling my armpit. Her sweet face brought an immediate smile to mine. Coffee cups, pajamas, and granddaughters playing eased us into the new day. We managed breakfast and then turned to arrangements for Phil's memorial service.

Beth suggested that we not have Reverend Van Dyke come out to the river to talk with us, but rather that we all go together to church the next day. She wanted to check out the facility and direct the flower arrangements. Heidi concurred; she wanted to inspect the reception room. House of Hope Presbyterian Church was my church, not theirs. Though they'd attended Sunday school there as children, only Jena had developed an ongoing closeness with a church community. I was grateful that her sisters wanted to reacquaint themselves with the church building. I called the pastor, who easily agreed to the Tuesday morning meeting at church.

That settled, we went to the mortuary, where we collectively wrote Phil's obituary, chose his urn, and set the date and time for his service. I cast the decisive vote for a Saturday service to give us time to prepare and to allow out-of-town folks to arrive and working folks a chance to attend. I knew I could not speed my way through executing the service as a task. I needed time to create a meaningful celebration of Phil's life.

That night we sat around my kitchen table trying to imagine hymns and instrumental music for the service. I was the only one who really understood how music could fill the House of Hope sanctuary with beauty, but I did not own a hymnal. Our family had no musical talent or training to draw on, but I'd saved the names of a few pieces performed at church that I particularly liked. The children turned to YouTube to explore other possibilities. In the end, we had a short list of suggestions to take to David.

As we entered the church library on Tuesday morning, my cell phone rang. The caterer I hoped to use for the reception was returning my call: she was available on Saturday. That was a relief. David invited us to sit around the big library table. Heidi immediately admitted to one and all that the church made her uncomfortable. She said, "Beth and I are good at logistics, though." Jena, a seminarian, was helpful in offering scripture ideas. As we told stories about Phil, only Chris lost his composure. The youngest child, he had had more of Phil's time than his sisters, but he lamented that he hadn't taken his dad up on more of his offers to do things together. "Maybe I should have tried hunting," he said softly.

I told everyone that I would like trumpets, Mozart, a soloist, and family speakers if anyone cared to volunteer. I gently warned David that I did not want to be portrayed as some kind of a saint in caring for Phil. He listened to all of us and steered us into a shared vision that allowed the music director independence in building on our wishes, that allowed David to create the order of worship, homily, and program, and that allowed me to turn over all management issues. He led us in prayer and set us free for lunch on Grand Avenue.

As we seated ourselves for pizza, I found myself facing a brightly tiled wall that appeared to represent the embers in their large pizza oven. Long ago Phil and I had chosen cremation for ourselves. On this day of his cremation, looking at that wall, I shivered. I closed my eyes and pleaded with God for Phil's spirit to be safely risen. I said nothing about my inner turmoil to the children. I was glad to get home.

The family scattered on errands. Abby and Ken came out to see me, bringing food and some wine from their recent trip to California. Retelling Phil's final days and the plans for Saturday's service, I felt their abiding love for us. Abby had been miserable in their absence, unable to come quickly and say good-bye to Phil. I couldn't begin to count all the times she and Ken had been there for us. I relied on their enduring friendship and told them I would need them even more when the family departed.

That night we enjoyed Sandy Kiernat's homemade chicken potpie. Over dinner, Chris agreed to read at Phil's service, choosing the Hopi prayer that reminded him of his dad, "I am the diamond glints on the snow." Jena felt she wanted to say something, without knowing yet what it might be. I said I thought I'd like to say something as well. After Beth put her girls to bed, she considered her part. She decided to read Mary Richardson's poem "The Heritage." Heidi did not want to address the congregation. I told her, "Your help over the long years of your dad's illness says more than words." David was lumping us together as "Family Remembrances" in the church program. Our plan could be fluid.

On Wednesday I retreated to my thinking room and gave myself the gift of writing. I wanted to hold Phil in my hands and give my heart a chance to express itself before the bustle of extended family arriving on Thursday. The children lovingly gave me my space. Words flowed. When the printer expelled the pages of my remembrance, I felt whole. Having reclaimed the goodness in Phil's life despite Alzheimer's, I tenderly folded the pages and set them aside for Saturday's service.

I recounted the time on board the *Argonauta* when we went under the Prescott Lift Bridge backwards. Losing control without mishap had been an exhilarating experience. In much the same way, losing control to Alzheimer's was not always bleak. In the early years, when we would set aside our plight and embrace what we could do, fun remained quite possible. I cherished our Lindblad trips. I saw Phil kneeling on the forest floor to examine tiny chocolate lilies, pressing himself against the rail to spot gray whales breaching, and soaring above the clouds to witness Denali in full sunshine. I even loved his occasional exasperation with the naturalists. "Their stuff is coming at me like bowling balls!" he had complained. Nevertheless, his capacity for delight in what he saw through his own lens had been in full force. I remembered our lovely dance in Wellstead's sunroom, when Phil gave no thought to where we were as he led us in graceful twirls and dips.

It was important to me to speak of our family during the long voyage with Alzheimer's. I wrote:

> Suffering from Alzheimer's coincided with one of Phil's greatest sources of delight, being a grandpa. At age six, our oldest grand-daughter, Madeline, may have diagnosed his illness the earliest. She explained proudly to one of our friends, "Grandpa is a rare bird, like a cardinal that says cock a doodle doo." Several years later, just after the Alzheimer's diagnosis, Phil and our oldest grandson, Max, were working in the yard together. Grandpa accidentally cut down a healthy young tree. When I came upon them, Grandpa was placing the rootless trunk in a bucket of water, presumably to grow new roots. Ten-year-old Max cautioned me to silence, say-ing, "Gigi, don't take Grandpa's hope away." His natural wisdom gave me hope that we would all find a way to honor Phil without allowing Alzheimer's to get in the way.

I purposely included every grandchild in my remarks because I wanted all of them to feel their importance to both Phil and me. Their loving acceptance of him had meant a lot. Phil's decline had been particularly hard for Max and Mimi, who had enjoyed Phil as the active grandpa he was meant to be. I deeply appreciated how our children had included their children in Phil's journey. We all had learned to face his difference with grace.

Heidi hosted supper and story night on Friday for twenty-two fam-ily members. Expectant grandchildren set up a poster emblazoned with a huge heart to receive our individual hearts after we each told a story about Grandpa. Dessert awaited each storyteller when his or her heart was placed inside the big Grandpa heart. There was no pressure to tell a story, but there was motivation! Everyone participated.

Heidi started by explaining how the heart activity was to work. She was candid that she was mad at Alzheimer's for stealing the last years of her dad's life. Jena recalled Grandpa making snow tunnels with Max and Mimi long ago and acting like a happy six-year-old himself. Beth reminisced about her summers working in her dad's office, recalling how the staff and patients loved him. It was her dad who surprised her with a puppy after months of begging him. Chris was amazed by his dad's ability to connect quickly with anyone in a friendly manner, always putting others at ease. I told about Grandpa's and my first kiss in a canoe that nearly swamped. Allie talked about her big brother who always looked out for her, except when he tried to beat her in sports.

The cousins had fond memories of coming to the river. Sarah, in particular, remembered Uncle Phil in his scrubs, whether on the way to the hospital or to cut down trees, always working so hard. Max and Mimi recalled trips to Florida where they enjoyed putting contests for Dairy Queens and learning to kayak. Max liked relaxing on the porch with Grandpa's orchids. Mimi liked to ride with Grandpa on his Minnesota tractor. Heidi's children wished they'd known Grandpa better. Walt, especially, knew that he and Grandpa would have been buddies. Cait and Imogen danced to Jane's guitar playing, showing how they were with Grandpa.

Sons-in-law Rob and Oliver told stories new to me. Rob met Phil on the ice, playing hockey. He wondered with amusement what this man, who would become his father-in-law, must have thought of him when he fought another guy who had bumped their goalie. Oliver saw Phil through his mum's eyes, with Phil genuinely wanting to answer her medical questions and respecting her as a nurse.

Afterwards Heidi would not allow us to help with cleanup; she sent us home for a good night's sleep before Phil's service. Neither Allie nor I slept well, however. The church celebration was so important to me: I needed to be lifted up by fine music, sacred text, and serene sanctuary. I wasn't worried about our program, any of the players, or the public, but I felt the finality to come.

When Heidi's family and I sat down in the front pew and the soloist sang Mozart's *Laudate Dominum*, I drew amazing comfort from the surrounding beauty. My heart melted, and then it soared with trumpets playing Pachelbel's Canon in D. Pastor Van Dyke gave the invocation and invited the congregation to sing "Joyful, Joyful, We Adore Thee." We continued in unison by reading Psalm 23. Fifteen-year-old Mimi confidently read Timothy 4:6–8 for her grandfather: "I've fought the good fight!" David then read Romans 8:18–39, which addresses injustice, human incapacity, and, still, promise. He referenced Kushner's *When Bad Things Happen to Good People*, saying we'd played the hand we were dealt with grace. Alzheimer's had definitely been a bad deal. Then he retold old family stories that brought back Phil in his prime. I loved listening.

Our family remembrances gave further dimension to Phil. Chris began, "I'm Chris, Phil's son." How grateful I was for that fact! I was able to read my piece with composure. Jena spoke from notes, highlighting her dad's unique way of doing things but also expressing how old tangles melted away in these years with chronic disease. Living in the moment was all that mattered and all that was possible. Beth closed by reading Richardson's poem, which spoke of the "great heritage of remembered joy" and proclaimed love binding forever. Young Walter's tears streamed. I put my reassuring hand on his long slender leg, hoping he would come to accept the release of his grandfather as part of life's cycle.

I closed my eyes to listen to the soloist sing "Shall We Gather at the River," so appropriate in layers of meaning. Congregational singing swelled in "Amazing Grace." Finally David blessed us all before we departed with Phil alive in our hearts. I trusted God to be faithful and present to Phil in heaven and to us as we carried on.

In the following weeks, condolence cards continued to pour in. David sent a CD of the service. I waited to play it until daylight faded. Sitting alone in my sunless sunroom, I welcomed the refreshing tears that finally came. A different night I taught myself how to make a photo book on my computer and created a volume in tribute to Phil. I typed up special messages that friends had written on cards. I inserted fifteen pages of them into folders for each of the children along with David's homily, our family remembrances, and copies of the CD of the service. I mailed copies of the photo book and the memory folders to the children and Phil's sisters, and to my mom and Phil's stepmom, who were not with us. For me, all the words brought Phil back to life in many different and wonderful ways. I began to peel back the Alzheimer's years and to enjoy the lively fellow who was my husband. Snowstorm after snowstorm buried me in the house, and I didn't care.

In time I did come out. My neighbor got me outside to enjoy walks in the winter wonderland. I drove into town for an overnight with Abby and Ken. Then I flew away to Florida to walk the beach and play golf with high school women friends, Joanna and Susan Gunderson from Boston. Over the years we had shared many adventures as couples. Revisiting those good times felt great. Susan thought to ask if I minded talking about old times. "They raise my glad quotient," I told her.

Back home in early March 2011, I wrote in my journal:

> So, dear Phil, you have been gone a month. You are no less a part of my life in your absence. I no longer hold your hand or see your eyes connect to mine, but I thank you for partnering with me to open so many doors to life over all these years. I trust I have more to open, but you will always be part of me as I do so. Perhaps I too am with you in your new home with the husk of our imperfections discarded and the essence of our delicate natures retained in some new way. God bless you, my Philly. Though it appeared that you lost all capacity to care and consider my well-being, I hope now that you know that I'm all right, unafraid, and eager to carry on. May some of your delight and determination fuel my future.

My Christmas present from Heidi's family was an invitation to join them that March on their trip to the Bahamas. As it turned out, I did not have to worry about Phil in our absence. I relaxed into their loving consideration. One day the boys caught fresh lobster, grouper, and snapper. "Gigi, get your camera!" Tom yelled from their boat. I was delighted to see and record their catch. I couldn't help thinking how excited Phil would have been to be part of the catching. Still, I reminded myself that my pleasure was no less for thinking about all the earthly things that Phil was missing. In addition to being with family, I savored the aqua waters, pink sand beaches, the largest full moon in twenty years, and my first green flash sighting.

When I came home this time, my short script of thanking friends and breaking away in travel was complete. Immediately certain of Phil's peace when he died, I had felt peaceful too. Now irrevocable loss and absence weighed on me. I'd been happy going places, sharing time with loved ones, and even cleaning out my garage, but I knew it was time to quiet myself and embrace the solitary serenity of my home. I wanted to turn off the voices of others and go inside myself. I felt called back to writing and the special time it gave me with Phil and the mystery of our life together.

I could not answer my own call, however. Mother fell ill in April 2011.

Beth, her girls, and I were visiting Texas shortly after Mother's ninety-ninth birthday. She collapsed at the breakfast table mid-sentence. Her mouth went slack, and her eyes dimmed. I held her in my arms, rubbed her back, and tried to arouse a response. Before the paramedics arrived, she came to and said she needed to throw up. She was surprised that we'd called for help and flustered to have created an ordeal.

She ended up in the hospital. Her regular doctor was away. The new fellow ordered lots of tests and frequent blood pressure monitoring. The net effect was that Mom's fear escalated. The doctor extended her stay in the hospital. Mom grew weaker, requiring two aides to help her on frequent trips to the bathroom. When the regular doctor returned, he read all the tests and came to the conclusion that Mom had simply fainted, most likely as a result of exhaustion from her bronchitis that had kicked up. After five days in the hospital she went home with her longtime aide and a new nighttime helper in place. I soon went back to Minnesota, hoping for Mom's usual recovery.

Several days later, she experienced another fainting episode. My brother, Ted, needed to go out of town on business, so I returned to Texas. The night helper had not worked out. I slept on a comfortable air mattress on Mother's floor, rather like the faithful family dog, to assure that she could get to the bathroom if she woke up. The arrangement could not be a long-term solution.

Mother seemed to grow stronger over a week's time. Her aide and I took her to the doctor's office for a checkup. His upbeat attitude instilled some confidence that Mother needed. I flew home again, still expecting Mom and her aide to come north for the summer in several weeks.

Then came another call. Mother had had a heart attack and was back in the hospital. I flew immediately back to Texas. Mother was experiencing hospital deliriums like Phil had when he shattered his pelvis in 2003. I could scarcely bear her fright, confusion, and despair. This was no way for her to go. I thought, "If only her breakfast-table collapse had taken her, then she would not have to suffer so." The doctors were recommending a pacemaker. I wasn't sure, but my brother and I ultimately agreed to proceed. Mother was in no shape to make the decision herself.

The procedure went smoothly, and Mother was transferred out of ICU to a quieter room, which basically meant less attention. I slept in a chair beside her bed. The doctor agreed with me that Mother needed to leave the hospital as soon as possible and get home to a familiar environment. We hired around-the-clock staff to be on deck and ordered an ambulance to take her home. "Mom, you will never have to go back to the hospital again," I promised. She was certain she would die before she reached Ted's ranch, but she did not. She entered hospice care at home, tethered to an oxygen tank.

She had lost her pluck, but Mother wanted neither to die nor to be an invalid. She ate chicken soup, generally cooperated with all the new helpers, and slowly regained some strength. We both knew, however, that her summer trip to Minnesota was in jeopardy.

Ted sent me home. He didn't want me to miss the writing camp I'd signed up for on Madeline Island. He understood that I needed a break from caregiving and a chance to be on my own for a while. Mother's health crisis on top of Phil's death had me running on empty. On my last day in Texas, Mother and I spent the morning outside. I pushed her wheelchair around the horse paddocks, dragging the oxygen cylinder behind. Before departure, I lay on the bed with her and rubbed her back for two hours. The quiet time of soothing touch calmed both of us. Occasionally she'd ask, "Is it time for you to go to the airport now?" She seemed to luxuriate in the response, "Not yet." When we parted, there were no tears. In a way, my leaving was a sign that she was better.

Breathing in fresh Lake Superior air on the ferry crossing to Madeline Island, I was grateful to be alone with my feelings and talents. I had not seen my writing coach, who would be leading the five-day retreat, for a long time. I didn't know how experienced the other writing hopefuls would be. I was not intimidated. I just wanted to listen to my soul and discover my voice. My favorite part of the time away was sitting alone at a picnic table with the sun on my back and notebook and pen in hand. A sandhill crane family with two chicks darted in and out of the tall grass unconcerned with my presence. Then the chicks disappeared, probably victims of a predator. Seemingly I was not meant to escape the consideration of death.

I returned to Texas in late June for a family meeting. Ted and I agreed in advance that Mother's seasonal transitions between Texas and Minnesota were likely over. The big question was where she should live out her days. Palliative home care and love was readily available in either state. Ted or I could travel back and forth on regular visits.

Our heartfelt discussion with all the pros and cons and assurances left the final decision to Mother. I actually feared her obvious anguish might cause another heart attack. The next morning, when I was helping her out of bed, she slumped forward and blurted out, "Your father would tell me to stay put!" I agreed, "It's probably the right thing to do." Then I heard myself offer, "Maybe you could just come for two months." Deep down I knew the prospect of forever was maybe more than I could handle. Mother brightened with the idea of a holiday in Minnesota, quickly asking, "Do you think Ted would go for it?" Like me, he softened his resolve. He told her, "If that's what you want and it's too much, then at least you'll die happy. But I'm telling you one thing, Mother: you are not going back to Minnesota for Christmas!" The deal was sealed.

There was one catch. Jena, Max, Mimi, and I were going to the Galapagos Islands for a week. We'd been looking forward to the adventure for over a year; the trip was prepaid, nonrefundable, and set for the last week in July. Heidi and Beth were ecstatic that their beloved grandmother was coming to Minnesota and vowed to pitch in while I was gone. The prospect of a Roy woman team was ambrosia to Mother. I reminded her that I was going to hire a full complement of staff too. "Whatever you want," she beamed.

I transferred hospice care to Minnesota, interviewed home health agencies, ordered a motorized bed, and collected Mother from Ted's care at the airport in mid-July. Beth and her girls were already in residence to cheer Gram on. The demands of Mother's care and the schedule of helpers she didn't want fell into ragged routine. After a week, with Beth glad to be in charge, I left for vacation a hemisphere away.

I hadn't known when Phil would die, and I didn't know when Mother would. She didn't intend to give up while she could enjoy her family. The hospice nurse thought Mother was doing remarkably well. Beth and Heidi were ready to face all eventualities. I would be too far away to do anything except enjoy myself. On a small ship in the middle of the ocean, there would be no getting back.

Meeting Jena and the grandkids in Miami, I broke into tears. Our long-imagined trip together was really happening! Jena gave me a big hug, and Max's and Mimi's alarm dissipated with my croaked question, "Have you seen happy tears before?"

We dove in, literally. Lone, agile sea lions would surprise us, darting close and disappearing in underwater somersaults. Dozens of yellow-tailed surgeonfish swam in smart formation, moving in perfect unison. Both the playfulness and the precision reminded me of Phil. He had been gone for six months, but I felt his enthusiasm and curiosity accompanying us on our expedition. Instead of missing him, I appreciated the family adventure that included his spirit. We were up early to hike the islands in search of wildlife. Hugely appreciative of Phil having introduced me to the natural world, I was thrilled to share that pleasure with two more generations.

Once I was back in Minnesota, August was a nightmare. Mother's happy spirit disappeared. Nothing suited her. As I tried to assist her in getting ready for bed, she pushed me away, "Nothing matters. Will you let up!" She refused to eat or to get out of bed for four days at a time, enduring hygiene care in place and mostly sleeping. Ted came to Minnesota. We consulted with the hospice nurse. Mother's vital signs were good. The nurse told us that vacillating mood was not unusual. The hospice doctor changed medications, and I was instructed how and when to administer them. I hated being in charge of what were called comfort medications. I felt more like Dr. Kevorkian than an angel of mercy. If Mother was sleeping, the medication often spilled out of her slack mouth. If she happened to be awake, she would push my hand away.

Heidi took my place sometimes, but I felt the unrelenting responsibility of providing Mother with whatever might help her without knowing what that might be.

I thought about Dr. Holm telling me that I needed to be Phil's wife again. I wanted to be Mother's daughter again. Aides sat in her room around the clock in eight-hour shifts. They would call me when Mother woke up. I checked on her frequently anyway. One morning she opened her eyes and said to me, "I love you." There had never been a question that that was true. Later, she told me, "I'm done. Good-bye." But dying wasn't that simple. Mother was frustrated with death's mysterious course. "I'm tearing out your heart!" she wailed. I told her that I loved her so much and was willing to suffer the heartbreak of losing her. "You are the best mom ever. Everyone knows it. You've taken such good care of us!"

Jena and Chris were coming to Minnesota for my birthday on August 19 and to bring love to Mother. She didn't want them to see her in her puny condition and began another five-day sleep. Miraculously, she woke up in time for cake in the kitchen. She even laughed, telling old family tales with Jena. She queried Chris, "Are you getting married?" He hugged her and said, "Stay tuned." It was such an unexpected, sweet time!

After her grandchildren left, I was quite certain that Mom's next effort to die was producing material results. Once again she refused to eat and withdrew. Continuing to administer the prescribed medications, I felt like an amateur scientist messing around with explosives. It was awful. I called Ted with an update, advising him, "I don't know if Mom will even know you, but you might want to come for yourself." We agreed to talk daily.

Lo and behold, the next day Mother woke up with renewed zest. The hospice nurse came. Mother's blood pressure was in the healthy range; her lungs were clear. Heidi and I were dumbfounded! I suggested to Mother that we call Ted. She did not express her usual worry that she would not be able to hear over the phone. He told her he'd visit in a few weeks while I went to Joanna's cabin for my fall women's retreat. Mother took in that news with equanimity. When Beth telephoned, Mother was very chatty, wanting to hear all the California stories. She told Beth, "It's getting cold in Minnesota, so I'll be going back to Texas soon." That was news to me. She'd not been out of her bedclothes in five days.

Happy hallucinations followed. Mother enjoyed what she saw, and I entered into the fabrications with her. One time she looked at me and exclaimed, "Here's my grandmother." I leaned over and kissed her, whispering, "I love you the best." Mom grinned, "I know." All my life she had told me stories of her grandmother who loved her best.

Heidi came faithfully nearly every day to see how we were doing. She agreed with the hospice booklet that the medication dance is impossible to understand fully, that the elderly metabolize medications poorly, and that many changes to medications, while well intended, mostly add to the uncertainty of what they are accomplishing. One day Mother would be scared; the next day she wasn't. Change was the only constant. Wishing for her to feel the reassurance of and confidence in God's presence, I posted Julian of Norwich's prayer in her room:

> The light of God surrounds you
> The love of God enfolds you
> The power of God protects you
> The presence of God watches over you
> Wherever you are, God is
> And all will be well . . .
> All manner of things will be well.

The words tenderly reminded me that I was not in charge.

In a lucid moment in early September Mother asked me, "Where did August go?" It was hard to explain. In private, the hospice nurse reiterated to me, "A roller-coaster ride toward death is not unusual." I thought about Phil's slow, mindless slide into eternity. Mother seemed to be doing a final cha-cha, dancing to a surprise beat. Again, her vital signs were perfect. She asked the nurse what she could do. "Anything you want," was the reply. Mother hesitated for a moment and announced, "I want to go to the Mall of America and eat tempura shrimp at Tiger Sushi." I'd been cleaning up her poop for two days and writing her eulogy while she slept. I declared nap time before we went anywhere.

When Mother woke up an hour later, she had not forgotten her lunch plan. The aide helped me get Mother dressed and into the car. With her transport chair in the trunk and fresh paper pants and her "do not resuscitate" paper in my purse, we three set off. We rolled into the mall about two thirty and suffered no wait at the restaurant. Sitting at a high bar table, I kept my arm around her so she wouldn't fall off the tall chair from which her legs dangled like a baby in a high chair. She could only eat half her lunch. In my nervousness I ate the other half plus my own.

As we exited the restaurant, Mom said, "Don't yell at me." I told her I was not yelling. "You'll yell when I tell you I want to stop in Nordstrom," she replied. We'd made it safely through the meal. Mother had now been up longer than she'd been in a week. Her bowels were on good behavior for the moment. How long could we stretch this adventurous moment? I didn't know if she was testing my patience, her luck, or the power of retail therapy. What she wanted was to buy me a birthday present. Reluctantly I steered her to a coat I'd been considering, put it on for her approval, and quietly told the Nordstrom sales clerk to ring it up posthaste. Garment bag in hand, Mother was satisfied. Once we returned home, she was asleep in ten minutes, genuinely thrilled by her moment of normalcy. I was exhausted!

When Ted came for the weekend, I thanked him and left immediately for Joanna's cabin. I'd been on call night and day for six solid weeks during which Mother appeared to be dying three different times. My retreat friends adored Mother and wanted to hear all the stories. She was the last of our mothers, and they savored her staying power. The mall story had them in fits of laughter.

I knew Mother's rally was tenuous at best, but I was delighted to see her spirits pick up. In my absence, she and Ted actually talked about her return to Texas in time for his birthday at the end of October. Much like the goal to get to Minnesota in July, this new goal gave her purpose. She sustained her rally. Beth flew in from California to share in the miracle. Indian summer weather prevailed. I moved ahead with the flight reservations for Mother, her aide, and me to fly back to Texas in the weeks ahead. As challenging as Mother's Minnesota holiday had been, I was glad we'd taken the chance to do it. She hadn't died, and she hadn't always been happy, but she'd received a lot of love.

Mother had been forced to resign herself to having a lot of helpers. In Texas Ted and I put a new team in place and reinstituted hospice, including a daily nurse to handle medications. Mother was grateful for her time in Minnesota and determined to release me with a brave face. She knew I would return to her, but there was no grand plan for her to pin her hopes on. She also knew she likely would never leave Texas again.

I was eager for the serenity of my own home minus the trappings of Mother's hospice care. Maybe I could answer that old call to go inside myself and explore how I was really doing. In the past six months, thoughts of Phil and even myself had been run over by the immediacy of Mother's needs.

The first Sunday in November was All Saints Day at House of Hope. The Motet Choir joined the Bach Chamber Players of Saint Paul to perform the cantata *Lux Aeterna* by Morten Lauridsen. As I listened and tried to keep place with the sung Latin and English translation, I gave up after "Grant them eternal rest, O Lord, and let perpetual light shine upon them." I allowed the music to fill me with Phil's nearness. When Pastor Van Dyke began to read the names of the deceased members of the congregation, I didn't know if I could bear it. Each name was followed by a soft gong. I recognized Jessie Bockstruck, John Davis, and suddenly the alphabet was at dear friend Glenn Stratton. I had been silently saying Phil's name over and over and filling with tears. Had I missed its reading? No. Greeting David afterwards, I whispered, "You accidentally forgot my Phil, but I did not!" I felt like the rung gong, vibrating with remembrance and wordless prayer.

The final hymn was "Fairest Lord Jesus," a familiar old song from my childhood in the Congregational Church. The second verse, "Fair are the meadows, Fairer still the woodlands, / Robed in the blooming garb of spring; / Jesus is fairer, Jesus is purer, / Who makes the woeful heart to sing," reunited me with my own woeful, childlike heart. I exited quickly to the privacy of my car and came home to my meadow and woods, thankful to have sung grief's release.

# CHAPTER 21

∧◻◻◻◻∧

# Grieving and Carrying On

Chris and Amber's engagement party was on Friday 11/11/11 in her hometown of Yankton, South Dakota. I was thrilled for them and for my freedom to hop behind the wheel and make the six-hour drive from the Twin Cities in solitude. I was looking forward to meeting Amber's family and to giving congratulatory hugs to my son and his bride-to-be. Amber asked me to bring my signature salad and some champagne. I also packed Phil's five remaining Orvis champagne glasses for parental toasting. Inclusive fun beckoned.

Friday afternoon was unseasonably warm. We sat in the backyard to get acquainted. Amber's aunt had brought fresh halibut from Alaska. Her dad set up the grill for steaks. Grandma Dolly had baked a cherry pie, using the cherries Amber had picked in Montana. I relaxed into the easy informality and family affection.

The next morning Amber and Chris took me for a hike along the Missouri River. Their dog, Hank, sprinted forward and circled back, chasing squirrels and sniffing for birds. The river, the dog, the fresh air—all felt like home. Everything seemed right.

My brother, Ted, did not know where I was. Before lunch he called my cell phone, wanting me to know that Mother had asked him to promise to let her die. She was back in bed, refusing food and assistance to the bathroom. My heart went out to both of them. "Ted, Mom will not die quickly," I reminded him and myself. The agonies of August flooded back. Nevertheless, I waited until Sunday to drive home as planned. Ted was glad to meet me at the San Antonio Airport on Monday. We needed each other's support. Maybe death would be Mother's friend this time.

She never acknowledged my presence in the mix of the soft hum of helpers' voices. Her eyes were closed. The hospice nurse told me that Mother was doing her work. On November 21, 2011, her ninety-nine and a half years of loving presence came to an end. I had spent the final days brushing her wavy white hair as her head lay on the pillow. Fanned out around her face, her hair looked like rays of sunshine. She was our family sunshine, warming us with laughter and stories that she would tell on herself and recall about us. Wanting death's release for her had bought me refreshing tears in a rainbow time of thanksgiving and memory. When the mortuary staff took her body away, I picked up her pillow and took it to my bed. Hugging the satin-covered foam, I fell asleep.

I was not greedy wishing for more of Mother. I had had so much. Everyone had. To the end she delighted in hearing the details of Chris's engagement, Max's college plans, Cait's tennis lessons, and all other direct reports from her grandchildren and great-grandchildren. All of her loved ones mourned her death in Texas. Assembling Mother's far-flung tribe in Minnesota shortly after Christmas, we created a story night as we had for Phil. Ten-year-old great-granddaughter Susan summed up Mother's spirit, "She always made me feel like she was glad to see me."

At Mother's memorial service the next day, both Ted and I gave eulogies for our parents, who'd been a couple for over seventy years. My CEO big brother's voice cracked when he said, "To Mother, I was always her little boy." He spoke glowingly of Dad's integrity and leadership. I spoke of Dad's values, one of which was to have guts, which in his case meant to believe in oneself, to face difficulties, and to dream big. In Mother's troubled August, she had stared up at me and said, "You have guts!" With Dad's portrait on the wall looking down on both of us, I had taken her assessment of me as a compliment.

Now, amid the small congregation of family and Ted's and my old friends, I reminded everyone that Mother always said the last thing to go would be her tongue. When she and Dad had retired to Florida away from family, Dad called their bedroom "Gram's phone booth." She would place and receive family calls, elicit new stories from afar, plan a rendez-vous, and offer optimistic advice. Her life was all about loving connection.

I told the gathering about a special night before Mother went back to Texas to die. I'd knelt before her wheelchair so we'd be eye to eye. Not surprisingly, she began speaking. I told her honestly that I couldn't follow what she was telling me. Then, I added, "I guess that's not the first time." My extra comment struck her funny. Not one for silence, she launched into the nonsense tongue twister "Peter Piper picked a peck of pickled peppers." I joined in, and we repeated it over and over again with laughter. The spontaneous joy in just being together was a gift that she simply refused to allow to dry up.

Following the service, we all gathered in the Kirk Parlour. The win-dows looked into the Garth, where Mom and Dad and Phil were nestled under a dusting of snow. Weeks earlier, Heidi and I had taken Mom's and Dad's commingled ashes to church before the ground was frozen. Heidi had used the shovel to widen the burial site to accommodate their large urn. Using a knitted shawl that I'd made for Mom as a sling, I lowered the urn into place. As we sprinkled yellow sweetheart rose buds into the grave, I offered Mother's often quoted phrase, "The best is yet to come," and asked that it be so in heaven.

On New Year's Day 2012 each family group packed up and went to the airport at their appointed time. Heidi took Beth's gang first. I drove Jena's team and took them out for a quick lunch on the way. When I returned, Chris and friends were chatting and watching the Vikings lose on TV. Finally, after delivering Chris and Amber to the airport after dinner, I walked into my empty house. The emptiness was not entirely unwelcome. I needed some solitude in my own sanctuary to discover who I might be without Phil or Mother to tend.

Weeks later, approaching the first anniversary of Phil's death, I won-dered where grief was hiding. Mother's illness and death had absorbed most of the previous year. Turning to Phil in this tender time, I was shocked when a wicked dream kicked sleep aside. Without context, I was loudly yelling at Phil, "You bastard!" It was my voice, and he was the target. I'm not ordinarily profane. And poor Phil, dead as he was,

was in no position to defend himself. I felt awful. But there it was! I believed that I'd forgiven him long ago for the incidents of nonsense and misery that find their way into a long marriage. Why did I have to accuse him now in ugly rage? The truth is I hated being left without my partner, without his support, his laughter, and his loving touch. Grief is angry sometimes.

The dream recalled to me an ancient hurt during our working days. In despair, I had turned out of our bathroom and inadvertently faced a watercolor above Phil's bureau. In it, a handsome brown trout was alone in the shadow of a rock. I stared at it for a long time. I saw Phil in the fish: muscular, territorial, hidden, poised for the hatch to flow to him.

Stunned by the image of wild beauty, I couldn't hate that trout or Phil. Grace drew me out of my own sense of limitation. It occurred to me that there was a chance that I could lure Phil out of hiding. What I knew from fly-fishing was that catching him was not the important act. Rather, removing the small barbless hook, holding him in my hand, admiring him, and freeing him were what mattered most for both of us.

I've kept the watercolor of the brown trout. It's a tender reminder of my enduring need to forgive not just Phil long ago, but also myself and others as we come up short now and then. I believe that natural goodness shines deeply within all of us and reveals God's loving presence in creation. Neither mistakes nor fits of disappointment can erase that core part of us. Even with Alzheimer's Phil resonated to the goodness in others for a long time.

He and I never intended to forego fly-fishing, but I eventually understood that it was no longer a viable activity for us. It was too complex. Personal safety was a big issue. Phil's judgment was off. He literally could be in over his head quickly. In my journal, I lamented my circumstance:

> I feel like a mindless, plastic bobber, just holding a fishing line to indicate a strike. I want to be a fly fisherman, delivering the line to the right riffle and drawing my mighty trout in for an appreciative look. Or, I want to be a trout among trout, swimming and living

in natural community. Or, I'd even prefer to be the line, gracefully looping in hopeful connection.

I am glad my plastic bobber days are over. Instead I fondly remember fly-fishing with Phil. Our waders still hang in the garage as a tribute to our happy days in the stream.

Phil returned to me in a second dream. We were on a sailboat, tacking effortlessly in open water. I was standing on the bow studying the waves. It occurred to me that we should be wearing life vests. I turned to Phil, happy at the helm. I mentioned the life vests. He smiled and said, "You've denied me nothing." When I turned around, we were suddenly on a dam with roiling water. We plunged into the abyss. The boat did not splinter on impact, but the mast and rigging were torn away. Phil was gone. I was sitting alone in the stern of an empty hull. The current carried me to the master of the lock and dam, who made clear that no insurance would cover the damage. I asked myself how I could pay for this horrific loss—and woke up in a sweat.

I treasure Phil's words, "You've denied me nothing." They were an immediate balm to the tired question, "What more might I have done?" I'm not impaled on that thorn, but it has scratched me from time to time. In further reflection, I think Phil may have been looking past me and speaking directly to God. In either case, hearing his voice in a declarative sentence was great comfort after years of scant and unintelligible speech. Phil's affirming words assured me of his appreciation for the life he'd known, the goodness in his heart, and a readiness to move on.

The lock master may have meant that Phil's death was an act of God, or he may have been God reminding me that salvation is a matter of grace, not a paid-up contract. I listened in a state of shock.

My response of wanting to pay for damages seems strange. Had I not already paid in terms of the loss of plans that Phil and I had shared for our retirement years? I could not really repay our friends or ever be sure that I had done all that I might have on Phil's behalf. Loving each other had been costly in terms of personal sacrifice. In the last ten years of our marriage we had satisfied our vows of self-giving. Our strong egos had softened. Each in our own way, Phil and I gave and shared to the end.

Perhaps my final payment for the privilege of loving Phil is telling our story. If so, then I'm doubly glad.

Writing gives me another chance to hold Phil in my hands as well as to put words to the mystery of marriage. The dreams I had about love and marriage as a young woman were only hopes made of cultural expectation and limited imagination. The dreams I've come to rely on are important messages emanating from deep inside me. They call me to attention and whisper truth in my ear.

On the actual one-year anniversary of Phil's death, Abby, Ken, and I walked the fairways at Somerset Golf Course to visit the trees planted in Phil's honor. With little snow cover in forty-degree temperature, our steps were light. Close up, Phil's trees revealed their set buds promising leaves to come. Kissing the cold bark, I imagined their new season. In bright winter sunshine, we friends remembered the abundance of Phil's life. I felt more thankful than sad. Phil would never be lost to our family or the others he touched. The seeds of his being were securely

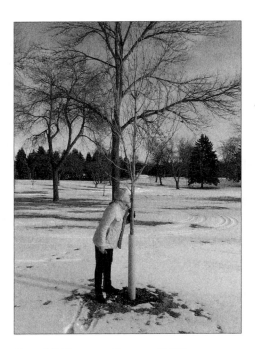

*One of Phil's trees on Somerset Golf Course*

planted in our hearts. We would be forever marked by his personality and love.

I couldn't go to sleep that night. Instead, I stayed up most of the night making a photo album of 2011. I'd never developed any of my snapshots during the year, but I had stored them on the computer. I worked from eleven at night until five in the morning before I pushed the send key, ordering a book for each of the children and me. What a year!

In 2012, without either Phil or Mother in my care, I was face-to-face with a new freedom. I picked up Jonathan Franzen's novel *Freedom* to lose myself in good writing and to explore a theme that had seemingly eluded me for a long time.

Much of the book's setting was a familiar St. Paul neighborhood. The family tensions between husband and wife, between parents and adolescents, between siblings, and between friends—all were plausible and wonderfully wrought. Each character struggled to figure out how to live in relation to freedom and choices. At one point, Walter Berglund, the dad, describes himself as "a purely reactive pinball in a game whose only objective was to stay alive for staying alive's sake." He imagined being a bird, not knowing what he knew and yet taking wing.

I would be dishonest to deny that I sometimes wanted to escape my caregiving role. I had not aspired to the job. Given it, however, I willingly accepted responsibilities, often experienced the feeling of being a pinball, and gladly cherished the blessings that filled my heart in the course of care. Now my caregiving role is done. There is nothing more I can do for Dad, Phil, or Mother. My choice of constancy feels right. Sprung free, I no longer wish to fly away. I'm happy in my nest.

The wonderful intermittency of special times with my children and grandchildren has not gone away. Phone calls, outings, trips, and emails keep us connected. I've even learned to text. I have more time for my friends. As executor, I have urged the estate work for Phil and Mother to conclusion. I look forward to the day when a truck comes to shred old files. Unlike story, the numerical records do not preserve their spirits.

This memoir has been a solace. My furtive attempt to patch together a story of Phil's life in 2005 recorded a bit of Phil's history for the family. This new story is about us and love's resilience and heartbreak. I sent a draft manuscript to each of our children, opening the window for their comments or concerns. Their response was illuminating to me. After weeks passed I casually inquired if my manuscript had been received. In their busy lives they had not carved out the right moment to dig into it. As Beth said, "Mom, it's not the kind of thing I would read at night and try to go to sleep." Jena perhaps spoke for all of them: "I have to be honest. The prospect is terrifying. I think of you as a private person." Their few words and larger silence have reaffirmed for me that this is my story. For better or worse, I'm free to do with it what I may.

In the spring of 2012 I was deeply touched that Phil's and my story found its way into one of my grandson Walter's entrance essays for St. Thomas Academy. With Walter's permission Heidi gave me a copy of his response to their questions, "Who is the person you admire most? Why?"

> The person I admire most is my grandma Barbara. She is my mom's mom. She has always been there when I needed her. But the thing I admire about her most is her ability to pull through anything. When I was four, my grandpa was diagnosed with Alzheimer's. My grandma was terribly sad and worked sleeplessly to help him, but still managed to be there as a grandmother.

I was astonished that this thirteen-year-old boy would think to hold up our Alzheimer's journey as an important lesson and claim my love for him as something he counted on. I was so proud of Walter for looking inside his family to articulate what was important to him. That he valued the ability to pull through anything and trusted me were huge in my heart.

Then, in August, I surprised the whole family and myself by throwing my own seventieth birthday party. I wanted to move past grief. Stuck with the big birthday, I decided to celebrate it. Actually the prospect of sailing into a new decade pleased me. My sixties had been all about caregiving. I was optimistic and curious about what my seventies might bring. I hired the Rockin' Hollywoods, who had played at my fiftieth high school reunion; invited lots of friends who'd stood staunchly by

Phil and me; and told my family they were off the hook for planning but not for dancing with me.

The day of the big event I suffered moments of doubt. What had I done? Ninety-three folks, many of whom did not know one another, invited for dinner and dancing? Then there was my dress: I had not tried it on since buying it in New York in March. Would it be too much? Also, there was my new eye makeup. My granddaughter Mimi had practiced putting it on me, but would it look out of character? And there were my new stiletto-heeled sandals. I knew from the test run in Dallas for Mom's birthday that they were not good walkers. Lastly, there was the band. I had enjoyed them at my class reunion, but this circumstance was different. This time I had the responsibility for directing them in setting the tone for merriment. The risk of being an old fool was real. Yet the potential reward of having a happy time with the people I loved most was appealingly possible.

The weather was spectacular, with no bugs. The food was excellent and the wait staff on the ball. Cocktail hour outside was lovely, save for my heels sinking into the lawn. Feeling like an oversized golf ball on a tee, I lurched about greeting guests. At seven, I had the band begin to play to draw folks inside. When nearly everyone was seated, the bandleader asked for the crowd's attention so I could greet them. I thanked everyone for coming, in particular the out-of-town guests. I said, "I hope you read the fine print on your invitations. This party is about celebrating the goodness of life. For me, that means family and friends. I could never have dreamed of the wonderful family that I have. And the value of friends in enriching my life is huge. So let's just have fun tonight. Thank you for being here for me. Enjoy your dinner, and prepare to do some dancing."

I had fun. I felt Phil wanting me to have fun. It was time for a party, a time for abandon and laughter, a time for merrymaking and dancing. As I'd hoped and imagined, it was over by ten p.m. All ages participated. And I was thrilled to survive being the center of attention without vanity tripping me up.

At summer's end, my house was quiet again. Writing resumed. At times I felt strangely shy and incompetent. Other times I churned out chapters in cathartic explosion. Phil's and my shared story was over, except for the writing of it. I wanted it on paper.

I took a time-out for my annual women's retreat at Joanna's cabin. Joanna had recently become engaged to a retired minister who lived on her lake. We were delighted for her, but that was nothing compared to her own giddy delight. John joined us on Saturday night to meet everyone, giving a good impression of quiet, deep water. Their wedding invitation asked poet Mary Oliver's question: "Tell me, what is it you plan to do / with your one wild and precious life?" Their response is to live it as husband and wife. I love their daring. May God bless them. For me, the thought of dating gives me the willies. I'm just getting used to living my one wild and precious life on my own.

# CHAPTER 22

# Being Me

Competing and doing one's best are part of the culture in which I grew up and from which I earned some sense of success. Playing fair and considering others were the rules of the road, but the system was far from perfect. Some folks rarely win, and some circumstances are unwinnable, as Alzheimer's was for us. Nevertheless, in this system, I'm counting on bright, hardworking scientists to figure out how Alzheimer's happens and how to prevent or counteract it.

Coming out as a loser was difficult for me. Uncovering me has meant claiming all my family support and admitting all my financial advantages. Few other caregivers are so fortunate. Though I experienced painful isolation before my husband entered residential care and heartbreaking challenges to the end, I cannot imagine being fully alone in the endless job. Some caregivers are. Many worn-out caregivers die before their loved ones do.

Phil's high-quality care did not erase the disease for him or for me. Alzheimer's is egalitarian, striking without regard to race, religion, gender, or means. The disease is a stark reminder to one and all: "It can happen to you." In addition, our four children face a factor that did not directly affect me. I was Phil's wife by choice; they were his children by blood. The ugly possibility that any of them might inherit Alzheimer's hangs in the air.

Many researchers use age sixty-five to separate early-onset and late-onset Alzheimer's. The greatest predictor of late-onset is simply age; the

older a person is, the higher the risk of getting the disease. Some researchers also divide Alzheimer's into familial and sporadic forms, which means
studying patients whose families include other members with Alzheimer's and patients who appear to be the only one with Alzheimer's. We
know of no other family members who'd suffered dementia. Deducing
that Phil belonged to an early-onset, sporadic group of patients did not
immediately explain how he came to have the disease or if the children
might have an increased chance of developing it.

Early on I was so preoccupied with Phil's pressing needs that I could
not immediately dig into the ghastly question of whether Alzheimer's
might also afflict some of our adult children in the future. By 2004,
when Phil and I went to the Mayo Clinic for a second opinion, I pressed
the hereditary question in private. I worried that asking about the children might make Phil feel horrible if he could comprehend that their
future problems might be tied to him. The professionals there could give
me no assurances or estimated odds about the children's health future.

All I could report to the children was that the Mayo doctors thought
the cause of Alzheimer's was some combination of genetic and envi-
ronmental factors in a complex story that they did not yet understand.
I am not a scientist. Despite being out of my depth, I reread and reread
the scant information on alleles in the Mayo book on Alzheimer's. Beth
had previously sent me a scholarly article from the University of Minnesota that addressed alleles in influencing Alzheimer's. I didn't know
what an "allele" is, and I still don't really. But the book said that an allele
called APOE e4 increased the chances of getting late-onset Alzheimer's
and quite possibly lowering the age of its onset. Essentially, not having
APOE e4 was better than having it. We didn't know if Phil had this
allele or if any of the children might have inherited it.

Heidi and Beth wanted to have Phil tested for the allele. If he tested
positive, they might decide to be tested themselves. They valued early
detection as a chance to seek early treatment, if it was available and
became necessary in their futures. Jena and Chris didn't want to know.
Their position emphasized living well in the current moment and not
worrying about the odds of Alzheimer's lurking in their futures. I didn't
know what such a test might entail. I didn't know how I might feel if I
were in their places. I assured them that there would be an autopsy at

Phil's death to measure relevant information, but while he was alive, I was going to concentrate on his care.

By the time Phil entered the nursing home in 2009, his cognitive capacities were nearly gone. I was sure he had no concept of his own illness or the possibility of passing it on to the children. I asked Dr. Holm about testing for the allele and found out a simple blood draw could be sent to a lab for such results. I told the children I was ready to request the test.

Reopening this issue was more important to Beth and Heidi, my scientifically oriented children, than to Jena and Chris, my philosophical ones. The philosophers supported the scientific siblings in their need to know but reiterated their desire not to know themselves. I wondered how a big secret would sit in the group, especially since I would have to know the results in ordering the test. Would my demeanor reveal what I would come to know? Would the sibling group become splintered somehow? Taking this step was a big deal for all of us.

Heidi helped me take her dad to Dr. Holm's office. Watching his blood being pulled into the tube, I saw scary, hidden, red truth. I asked Dr. Holm how many others of his families had requested this test. None had. Then I became alarmed, worrying that the test was so specialized and unusual that I'd signed up for a $10,000 procedure without realizing it. Checking, he said a few hundred dollars would cover the lab. He reminded Heidi and me that the results would not be definitive: having APOE e4 only meant an increased risk for Alzheimer's, not that the person would necessarily get it or not get it.

Weeks passed until Dr. Holm called with the results. I liked not knowing. I did not tell anyone outside the family what we were up to. If two of the children didn't want to know the answer, then I certainly didn't want any of my friends to know something my own children did not know. This was a private family affair. I tried to calm myself with the notion that the test didn't really matter, all the while devastated by the possibility that anyone else in the family might suffer Alzheimer's in the future.

The results loomed threateningly. I couldn't help my anxiety. The results mattered even if they were not "definitive." Dr. Holm took his time with me. I could barely listen to what he was saying. When I heard that the APOE e4 allele was not present, I yelped in relief. Phil didn't have it, so he couldn't pass it on to the children. I immediately called Heidi, blurting out the good news with the caveat, "You never know what I may have passed along." We both called Beth. They seemed satisfied that we knew what we could for the time being.

I couldn't leave Jena and Chris out. I called them as well to report that the nondefinitive test results were back and for what it was worth their dad did not have the risky allele. Jena laughed, perhaps with relief. She quipped, "I'm always glad to know that I don't really know anything."

Scientists are learning more and more about Alzheimer's, testing theories involving amyloid plaques and neurofibrillary tangles. They are studying inflammatory responses, oxidative stress, calcium levels and possible correlations between Alzheimer's and head injury, high blood pressure and cholesterol, and depression. Yet causes remain uncertain. And there's still no cure.

Losing one's mind is a fearsome prospect. I was a brainy kid who grew into a thoughtful adult. How could I be me without thinking capacity? Being smart not only had advantages in a meritocracy but was also the human capacity that allowed me to ask questions, to see humor, to tune to beauty, and to consider ethical matters.

Years ago, when I moved from public affairs to the trust division at U.S. Bank, professionals from Martin-McAllister Consulting Psychologists interviewed me. The Myers-Briggs assessment identified me as an INTJ, a rather rare personality type. I liked the idea of being somewhat of an oddball, different from others. The evaluation process concluded with a final report that was quite affirming. Under intellectual characteristics the report told me I was "exceptionally bright" and a "clear-headed thinker." Under emotional factors, it recognized my "self-discipline." Under interpersonal style, it noted "exceptionally strong leadership ability." I was particularly pleased to read, "You are a tough-minded individual who will face into problems directly and talk about them in straightforward ways." Lastly, under motivations the report correctly held up "intellectual curiosity," "spirituality," and "living according to particular values" as keys for work I deemed important. That I kept the report says something about my need for validation at the time and perhaps about my housekeeping since. Now twenty years later, I laugh kindly at my clever self who took a long time to notice Alzheimer's in our home.

Leaving the trust division and paid work behind, I became my own boss again in 1993. The first day I started up our tractor and cleared a new garden patch by our beach. The blade left naked roots sticking out of the sandy soil, so I turned off the motor and pulled out the remnants by hand. Sweaty from the hot sun and exercise, I happily wiped my hair out of my face and planted hostas along the embankment. Pleased with the project, I put away the equipment and headed to the shower. The hot water felt good until my skin began to tingle in a familiar way. I was covered in poison ivy. The bare roots had not been identifiable, but the itch was unmistakable. I agonized in physical and emotional defeat. It seemed at the time that I wasn't immediately smart at being in charge of myself.

In 1994 I began journaling, a practice I've kept ever since. The gift of writing has opened my eyes and heart in such life-affirming ways. At the end of the first year, I wrote in my new journal that I'd learned two things: I wanted to hear my own voice, and making sense of the world was less important to me than experiencing it.

Coincidentally in 1994 I became a grandmother, a life-altering and blessed experience. When the call came from Boston announcing the arrival of Max, Phil and I were ecstatic. Without Phil's noticing, I pinned a note on the back of his sport jacket that said, "I'm a new grandfather." Off he went to the hospital. I immediately booked my airline ticket east. The next day Jena and Max came home from the hospital, and a taxi soon delivered me to their back door. The explosion of feelings upon seeing them gave me an astonishing sensation of my own milk coming in. Max did not have to win my heart; he simply had it.

Max is now eighteen and a freshman at the University of Puget Sound in Tacoma, Washington. In October 2012, all eight of my grandchildren came to Montana for their Uncle Chris's wedding. Three generations celebrating together is such sweet song. With Mother gone, I am now the matriarch of the tribe, without prescribed responsibilities. I did ask Chris what I might do for the wedding. "Just come, Mom, and be yourself," he told me. What a lovely invitation!

The day before I left for the wedding, I made a pot of tea and sat at the kitchen table to write a poem for Amber and Chris. Writing a ditty

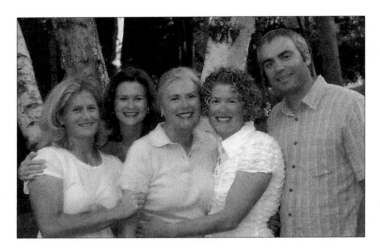

*Jena, Beth, me, Heidi, and Chris in 2009*

for special occasions is a usual practice of mine. I put key words, the alphabet, and letter blends at the top of the page. Using iambic pentameter, I jot line after line in rhythm and rhyme. It's a fun word puzzle that allows me to say something lighthearted and on point. Family and friends have grown used to my pleasure in offering these gifts of words.

I finished the wedding poem and tucked it in my suitcase. It would work as a toast, if toasts were to be given. On rehearsal night there were no toasts, so I left the two pages of verse under my dinner plate. At the wedding dinner, however, young people began to tell old stories and offer congratulations using the band's microphone. Jena, Heidi, and Beth stood together, as Heidi spoke briefly for all of them, "Welcome to the sisterhood, Amber!" I waited to see if Amber's folks would go forward, but they did not. Eventually, I did. On the way back to my place at the table, Amber and Chris stood to embrace me in thanks. Being myself felt right to me and evidently okay to them.

That I like words and am unafraid to stand up and use them is a part of who I am. I value being present not only to family but also to community issues. Being a member of the Wilder Foundation's board continues to connect me to the needs of folks who are not as lucky as I am.

Beyond services, Wilder also has a highly respected research division that focuses on vulnerable populations. Every three years Wilder

Research performs a statewide homelessness survey on a single day. Over one thousand trained volunteers conduct carefully crafted interviews of homeless individuals and families living in shelters, transitional housing, abandoned buildings, and known encampments outdoors. Public policy makers and service providers use the final homelessness report to monitor changes in homelessness and to improve the service system.

On October 25, 2012, I became an interviewer for the first time, knowing that there is a great deal of difference between believing in Wilder's mission of serving the poor, sick, and needy of St. Paul and actually sitting down together face-to-face. I was nervous. The thirty-six-page questionnaire seemed daunting to me, and I only had to ask the questions exactly as they were worded. Coming into the Union Gospel Mission for my four-hour shift, I couldn't immediately find the site coordinator and felt out of place in the men's emergency shelter operation. I didn't want to intrude. My good-hearted, hardheaded, able-bodied self was definitely out of its comfort zone.

On my own I found a windowless room with a carton of questionnaires sitting on the table and sat down to see what would happen next. Other volunteers and the young, cheerful coordinator showed up. He'd been successfully talking to shelter residents to ask them to volunteer for the confidential interviews. He gave me a questionnaire and soon returned with a resident. I chose to have us sit side by side at the table, not across from one another. I smiled hopefully, greeting him, on script, by giving my name and explaining, "We are doing a survey of people who do not have a regular or permanent place to stay. We would like your help. We are trying to collect information that will be helpful in creating affordable housing and planning other services."

Off script, I told him I was a volunteer too, but that I'd been trained to ask the questions precisely so the study would be done properly. He agreed that we could work together. I nodded encouragingly to him as I turned page after page in the interview booklet, marking the appropriate boxes for his responses. Asking about age and marital status was straightforward, but asking about things like jail time and sexual abuse was not easy. I tried to keep my tone even and nonjudgmental, but I couldn't help feeling that I was getting into his business. I admired his spirit when he looked at me and said, "I have nothing to hide." He wasn't discounting his pain. Rather, he appeared to enjoy helping me with the interview.

The men's stories varied. None of my interviewees was homeless by choice. Only one denied suffering from any mental health issue. A young man proudly told me, "I've been clean for three and a half months. My family wouldn't believe it." Then, smiling at me, he said, "I haven't had anybody to tell." Sharing his good news seemed to make him happy.

It was interesting to me that none of the fellows refused to answer any of the questions. After each interview, we returned to the auditorium to find the coordinator. "How'd she do?" he asked the resident light-heartedly. We always ended with handshakes and smiles. One gentle soul told the coordinator, "I never thought I could do anything like this before. I was too scared." I thought to myself, "There's been plenty in his life to make him afraid."

After my shift I walked into the cold night touched by the real men who would become statistics for possible change. In the process of my collecting Wilder's needed data, they had given me the privilege of see-ing into their hearts. I couldn't fix their situation, but I'd been present to them. Their raw vulnerability reminded me of Phil. Staring into the faces of homelessness and Alzheimer's, I felt weak.

What is life asking of me?, I wonder. For whom shall I care? About what shall I care? When do I play? How dare I be me?

# Acknowledgments

Loving support of family and friends kept me whole during the course of caregiving. Many of their names are in my narrative, but many are not. I carry in my heart all their kindnesses and tender words without which I might have withered.

Professional helpers at all levels gave us our best chance to live life fully. Again, all of their names are not in my narrative. That they continue to help others is good news indeed. Wayne Caron died unexpectedly while Phil was living at Wellstead. He encouraged me to say, "Ouch!" I am thankful that as a professor at the University of Minnesota, he trained many graduate students to carry forward his nationally respected work to serve families with a loved one suffering from dementia.

Organizations like the Alzheimer's Foundation are dedicated to care and services for individuals confronting dementia and also for their caregivers and families. I am particularly proud of the Amherst H. Wilder Foundation's Adult Day Health Program and Caregiver Resource Center in St. Paul, Minnesota. The affordable, integrated team approach consisting of nurse, social worker, occupational therapist, activity specialists, and primary care on site has been developed on evidence-based and/or research-based outcomes. The quality of life for individuals and their families can improve with effective support.

For me, faith is essential, though I was often too busy doing what I could do to rely on God. In testifying to grace, I admit my inadequacy to reveal profundity as it has touched me. Simply said, I have felt God's loving presence in both my caregiving and my writing.

In matters of writing, I thank first my freshman English teacher at Edina High School, Miss Costello. She taught me the art of writing a paragraph, a creative act that could be mine. Ever since then I've enjoyed putting words on paper. Most recently, I thank my writing coach, Elizabeth Jarrett Andrew, who lit a candle, gave me tea, listened, and encouraged me to write for myself. I thank my development editor, Beth Wallace, who pushed me to write a story for others. And I thank Beth Wright and Ann Delgehausen at Trio Bookworks, who believed in my capacity and desire to express myself and urged my book to publication.

Lastly, I salute the artists who directly helped me by their clear-eyed interpretations of life. Painter Edie Abnet understood the image and the importance of our Prescott Lift Bridge scene. Photographer Laura Crosby honored Phil and many other brave souls with dementia in her tender frames. And poet Anne Simpson gave me nuggets of truth in celebration of our tattered but nonetheless precious experience. Other writers, whom I do not know personally but reference in my narrative, spoke to me. Their honest words were gifts, as I can only hope mine may also be.

# Sources Cited

Bayley, John. *Elegy for Iris*. New York: St. Martin's, 1999.

Caron, Wayne A., James J. Pattee, and Orlo J. Otteson. *Alzheimer's Disease: The Family Journey*. Plymouth, MN: North Ridge, 2000.

Coste, Joanne Koenig. *Learning to Speak Alzheimer's: A Groundbreaking Approach for Everyone Dealing with the Disease*. Boston: Houghton Mifflin, 2003.

Crosby, Laura, and Anne Simpson. *"I'm Still Here": The Alzheimer's Journey*. St. Paul: PhotoBook Press, 2008.

Franzen, Jonathan. *Freedom*. New York: Farrar, Straus and Giroux, 2010.

Lamott, Anne. *Bird by Bird: Some Instructions on Writing and Life*. New York: Pantheon Books, 1994.

Mace, Nancy L., and Peter V. Rabins. *The 36-Hour Day: A Family Guide to Caring for People Who Have Alzheimer Disease, Related Dementias, and Memory Loss*. 5th ed. Baltimore: Johns Hopkins University Press, 2011.

Oliver, Mary. *New and Selected Poems*. 2 vols. Boston: Beacon, 1992–2005.

Petersen, Ronald, editor in chief. *Mayo Clinic on Alzheimer's Disease*. Rochester, MN: Mayo Clinic, 2002.

Simpson, Robert, and Anne Simpson. *Through the Wilderness of Alzheimer's: A Guide in Two Voices*. Minneapolis: Augsburg Books, 1999.